MW01194269

Live Better Longer

LIVE
BETTER
LONGER

*The Parcells Center Seven-Step Plan
for Health and Longevity*

Joseph Dispenza

HarperSanFrancisco
An Imprint of HarperCollins*Publishers*

HarperCollins Web Site: http://www.harpercollins.com
HarperCollins®, 🔥®, and HarperSanFrancisco™
are trademarks of HarperCollins Publishers Inc.
FIRST EDITION

Library of Congress Cataloging-in-Publication Data
Dispenza, Joseph.
Live better longer : the Parcells Center seven-step plan for health and longevity /
Joseph Dispenza. — 1st ed.
Includes index.
ISBN 0–06–251422–9 (cloth)
ISBN 0–06–251421–9 (pbk.)
1. Naturopathy.   2. Self-care, Health.   3. Health.   4. Longevity.   I. Title.
RZ440.D58   1997
613—dc21   96–39224

97 98 99 00 01 ❖ RRDH 10 9 8 7 6 5 4 3 2 1

*This book is affectionately dedicated
to the memory of*

Dr. Hazel R. Parcells,

*who labored a long lifetime to uncover
the healing secrets of nature.*

Contents

Acknowledgments

I would like to thank the many people who helped make this book possible.

Sebastian Puente and Ron Savarese, my colleagues at Parcells Center, whose vision, passion, and tireless energy have kept the important pioneering work of Dr. Parcells alive and made its message of hope available to the public.

Larry Martin, assistant and companion to Dr. Parcells for the last three years of her life, whose encouragement and technical knowledge contributed to the book in a fundamental way.

Judy Klinger, my research assistant, whose professionalism and enthusiasm added immeasurably to the project.

For their helpful advice and support, Snow Anderson, Dr. Samuel Berne, Vera Borgmeyer, Barbara Brennan, Les Brown, Julia Cameron, Mary Lou Cook, Dr. Joanna Corti, Debra Denker, Mary Kay and Joseph Del Priore, my father, Joseph Dispenza, Joyce, Stacy, and Michael Dispenza, Ursula Drabik, Jill Drinkwater, who introduced me to Dr. Parcells, Autumn Golden, Monica Faulkner,

Dr. Donald Frazer, Ben Galison, Ann Louise Gittleman, M.S., C.N.S., Burton Goldberg, James Gribble, Mark Hess, Alan Hutner, Hal Isen, Terry Kast, Daisy Kirkpatrick, Dr. Susan Lark, Ann and Lee Lefton, Richard Leviton, Dr. Jacob Liberman, Dr. Sabine Lucas, Robin McPeters, Richard and Rosemary Mead, Carl Miller, John Nicksic, Mary Savarese, Donald Sharpe, Tamar Stieber, James Templeton, Steve Thompson, Stephanie Train, Linda Turner, Dr. Gary Young, and Michele Zackheim.

Elaine Markson and her associates at the Markson Literary Agency, who extended every effort to bring the legacy of Dr. Parcells to light. And Caroline Pincus, my editor at Harper San Francisco, who saw the great value of this material and guided its framing and articulation with intelligence, understanding, and creativity.

To these and to the many former students of Dr. Parcells too numerous to mention, I am immensely grateful.

Foreword

In February 1974, a friend shared with me an advertisement she had cut out of *Let's Live* magazine. The ad promoted the Parcells School of Nutrition and promised "five days that would change your life."

And so, in February of 1974, my life was forever changed. I attended the Parcells School of Nutrition and was inspired to become a nutritionist devoted to the health of the people of this planet, armed with the incredible healing insights I learned from Dr. Hazel Parcells's many years of research and experience.

From the very first, I recognized her as a master healer and pioneer far ahead of her time. Her knowledge of color therapy, minerals, and the acid/alkaline balance of life opened new vistas of awareness in me. Her understanding of the underlying causes of disease in the twentieth century, such as parasites, heavy metals, and radiation, left me awestruck.

Nobody, but nobody, was teaching or writing or even thinking about such things in those days—yet now not a day goes by when the media does not bring an environmental issue to our awareness. Dr. Parcells said it would take about twenty years before mainstream Americans would question the purity of their water and the wholesomeness of their food supply . . . and it surely has.

Dr. Parcells's revelation that many people seeking true health will never get well until they rid themselves of parasites was a particular pearl of wisdom for me. After clearing my own system of both worms and amoebas, I incorporated the parasite connection to health into my own nutritional philosophy. In fact, I wrote a book called *Guess What Came to Dinner: Parasites and Your Health.* This book is dedicated "To Hazel R. Parcells, Ph.D., D.C., N.D., whose relentless search for truth and the underlying causes of disease inspired my life's work in the science of nutrition." Her practical day-to-day advice on the selection, preparation, and cleansing of foods with her famous Clorox® bleach formula was again put to good use, both personally and professionally.

My book *Beyond Pritikin* contains an entire section called "Chemistry in the Kitchen"—a concept I first learned from Dr. Parcells. I place special emphasis on the removal of all aluminum in the kitchen because of her statement, "In my kitchen, I would rather have the most deadly serpent than aluminum." To this day I shudder at the sight of aluminum foil, aluminum pots, and deodorants with aluminum in them.

I was particularly fascinated with her keen awareness of the devastating effects of radiation and fallout. Although we can't see it, smell it, or feel it, radiation is with us—and she warned us for years about radiation's immune-depressing and cancer-causing effects. Her salt and soda baths have become a matter of course for me after a plane trip or an X-ray treatment.

Dr. Parcells is indeed a legend. What I respected and admired about her the most was her ability to pinpoint the underlying causes of the health problems of our time and provide easy, natural solutions to remedy them.

This book is the bible of the Parcells Method—a comprehensive survey of all her unique and effective approaches to getting well, staying well, and living a long, full, happy life—according to the principles of nature.

Joseph Dispenza is a gifted writer on health. He writes with authority and conviction from deep wellsprings of knowledge. Here he not only explains all the profound mysteries of Dr. Parcells's work—and does it in a way that everyone can understand—but he also captures her remarkable personality, which has inspired so many of us who now labor in the service of better health for all people.

I know you will be as deeply moved by this book as I was. Its message is that we can take charge of our health and be well—and live long—if we have the information we need.

This book contains that information. And so much more.

Ann Louise Gittleman, M.S., C.N.S.
Certified Nutrition Specialist
Author of *Beyond Pritikin*

Introduction

The Extraordinary Dr. Hazel Parcells

Your eyes flutter open on the new day. You hear birdsongs calling up the dawn light. It is morning, and you feel good, alert, and ready for what today will bring. A smile breaks across your face. You stretch and yawn deeply, taking in the first breath of the day. It's like being reborn.

That faint smile greets you in the mirror. You go about your morning routine with a sense of well-being and the joy of anticipating what you will add to this day. You enjoy a wholesome and satisfying meal and go off into the world.

Everyone you encounter greets you with the same smile you saw in the mirror when you arose. You are pleasant to people because you truly like them. You are deeply centered, balanced, and happy. Work is done well and easily—it's almost like play. You feel good.

In the afternoon you take a half hour to be by yourself and go for a brisk walk. Your steps are lively as you reflect on all the fine people who help make up your life. That thought brings you joy and emotional nourishment.

In the evening you are still energetic, so you devote some time to family and friends. You say "I love you" to the people you love—and they return your declarations of affection. You eat a delicious meal and really enjoy it. Later, you spend an hour reading a good book.

As night comes on you feel blissfully sleepy. Preparing for bed, you remember the day and are glad for its pleasures and its lessons. Five minutes later you are enjoying a deep, satisfying sleep, from which you know you'll rise refreshed and replenished.

You are the picture of health.

It is a picture that can be a reality all your days. Well-being, in body, mind, and spirit, is your birthright as a child of earth. You are a part of nature—the thinking, reflecting part—and health should come naturally to you.

This was the picture held by Dr. Hazel Parcells, pioneer of nutrition and natural living, for sixty-five years—from the time she reclaimed her broken body from the ravages of an incurable disease in 1931 to her quiet passing recently at the age of 106. For Dr. Parcells, health was not an illusive goal, but a joyful way of living that brought day after day of full and gratifying well-being.

This book is her generous legacy to all of us who are seeking to live life completely, joyfully, and in good health.

Shortly after I moved to New Mexico from Los Angeles twenty years ago I began hearing about Hazel Parcells.

From accounts of people who knew her, I learned that she was a remarkable woman who had developed a unique form of self-healing based on many years of original research in nutrition. She lived in Albuquerque, where she taught classes and helped people regain their health. Her methods were extraordinary, they said, and her success with even terminally ill clients was nothing short of miraculous.

Whenever Hazel Parcells's name cropped up in conversation, the reports were always the same—amazing—and the urging to find her spiked with the same admonition: if I wanted to meet her, I'd better do it quickly, because she was, well, up in age. She was around eighty-five at the time.

Years passed. Every so often I would hear from someone who had heard from someone else that Hazel Parcells was the final authority on nutrition and naturopathy, and that I ought to look her up and find out about her unusual healing methods. The mention of her name was invariably accompanied by the caution about her advancing age. By then she was ninety-five but working vigorously and influencing new generations of health-conscious people.

More years sped by. Now and then I would be reminded that Hazel Parcells was still alive and, incredibly, still at work. She had turned 102 and was continuing her teaching and the application of her impressive research in natural healing.

When I finally decided to try to meet her, I had trouble finding her in Albuquerque. She had lived there for more than thirty years but had recently moved north to a remote valley nestled in the mountains about half an hour's drive northwest of Las Vegas, New Mexico. My first reaction was one of astonishment: I asked myself not only *why* a person who was more than a hundred years old would pick up and move into a new house in a new location, but, knowing the difficulties of moving at any age, *how* it could be done.

With two friends, neither of whom is a health professional—one is a stockbroker, the other a computer programmer—I drove one pleasant autumn Saturday morning to Sapello. It took longer than we had expected to get there, but we didn't mind because the scenery was magnificent and became increasingly more enchanting as we went farther up into the foothills of the Rockies. Suddenly I knew the answer to *why* Hazel Parcells would want to live up here. Compared with the teeming urban center of Albuquerque, the silence and the beauty of this place made it a natural paradise.

After all the years of listening to stories about her, I was prepared to encounter an interesting, but rather earnest, and certainly elderly, woman: she had celebrated her 105th birthday a month earlier.

The person who met us at the door with a wink and a wide smile, however, was neither solemn nor—much to our surprise—elderly.

"Well, hi, hi!" she said cheerfully.

She wore a bright red wool dress, which accentuated a freshly coiffed, full head of curly red hair. Her smooth cheeks were creamy pink, and her eyes twinkled with vitality. She was a diminutive Irish colleen. The cane in her right hand seemed more like a prop than a necessity, a concession to our idea of how a hundred year old should comport herself; when my eyes went to it, her face opened into a conspiratorial smile and she let out an impish laugh. I couldn't help but laugh along with her.

We sat in her living room and talked for the entire afternoon. Actually, *she* did most of the talking. She roamed intelligently and insightfully around in a surprising myriad of topics on the subject of health, from environmental illness to the politics of medicine to the latest discoveries in chemistry and physics. All of what she said was informed, and all of it related to the work she had been doing quietly over sixty-five years of tireless study.

It may have been my imagination, but at a certain point in the conversation she seemed to focus her attention on me and began speaking urgently about health and the future of the planet as if I were the only other person in the room.

When my friends and I left Sapello that evening, I was in a mild trance. The next afternoon I found myself up in the mountains again, this time alone. I parked at the turnoff to her long driveway for the better part of an hour, staring mindlessly at the modest rural mailbox that announced "H. R. Parcells," then turned around slowly and drove back to Santa Fe.

A week later I phoned for an appointment to see her and was told by her assistant, "Yes, by all means, come up. Dr. Parcells has been expecting you."

She indeed had been waiting for my return visit. She wore a smart, businesslike kelly green dress; around her neck hung two long strands of pearls.

We sat across from each other on comfortable couches and talked for several hours through that afternoon. Again, she did most of the talking. For more than half her life she had been a teacher, and that was apparent in the way she spoke to me—with authority, clarity, and a certain amount of drama.

"People are learning not only that they *should* start to take responsibility for their own health," she said, "but that, with a little good information, they *can* take on that responsibility."

She spoke from experience, I soon discovered. As a war bride during World War I she moved with her husband from Colorado, where she was born, to an army training base in Illinois. There, exposed to terrible weather and living in wretched sanitary conditions, she contracted tuberculosis. At the time, TB was as unconditionally lethal as the dreaded terminal diseases of our own day.

After the war she left her husband and returned to Colorado and worked at various jobs, pouring her deteriorating physical energy into, especially, cosmetology. By 1930, when she was forty-one, she owned and operated a successful beauty parlor—and used up all her business profits on doctors, each of whom held out a morsel of hope for her recovery. Recovery did not come, though. Her breathing became increasingly more shallow and the unremitting pains across her back more excruciating. She was weak from coughing, she couldn't sleep, and her skin had taken on a gray pallor.

Her condition worsened by the day. Early in 1931, she packed herself into her car with a friend, drove to Denver, and checked herself into Fitzsimmons Army Hospital, a renowned medical facility.

"The doctors took one look at me and shook their heads. I underwent a battery of tests, but they already knew I was near the end. I knew it, too. The X rays showed that my heart had become enlarged, that one of my lungs had collapsed under infection, and that I had hemorrhaged away a third of a kidney. My friend burst into tears."

As she spoke, her voice rose. She absently fingered her pearls, as if they were charms marking the infirmities she had suffered so long ago.

"The doctors gave me their verdict: I was going to die. They handed me a useless milk-and-eggs diet that was supposed to help keep me together for a time, and they offered to put me up in what they called a 'clinic'—it was a 'death house,' really. They told me there was nothing more medical science could do—and I believed them!"

Instead of enrolling in the Denver death house, she returned home and went back to work in the beauty shop. The next day, with death staring her in the face, she decided to do something life-affirming. She sat in one of the shop chairs and asked one of her employees to give her a luxurious color rinse and permanent.

"I didn't see my death sentence as final judgment, but rather as an opportunity. After all, the doctors had admitted there was nothing more they could do to save my life. Now my future was completely up to me."

She should have been depressed beyond consolation, but instead, as she related the story to me sixty-three years later, an exhilarating feeling of liberation came over her.

"I thought, well, I'm free to experiment and to try to discover something about how my body worked. One thing was certain—I wasn't going to get any worse. The first thing I did was to look at what I was eating. My eating habits had been awful. Because I was so ill, there were days when I wouldn't eat anything at all. I began to listen to what my body really craved and decided I would eat only that. Do you know what I wanted more than anything else? Something green. And the only green vegetable I could find at that time of year was spinach."

For months she ate practically nothing but spinach. She ate it fresh in salads, steamed, in soups. When she woke in the morning, she drank glasses of spinach juice. In a few weeks she was buying spinach by the gunny sack and using it up as fast as she could get it into the house.

The "miracle" began to happen shortly after she embarked on the spinach regime. Her energy improved a little, her back pain lessened, then her coughing bouts subsided. She was able to get through a night's sleep without waking up soaked in perspiration.

"Three months after I had been given my death sentence, I was starting to feel almost normal. After six months, still eating my spinach and other green vegetables like parsley and asparagus, I was a new person. I went back to Fitzsimmons for a physical examination a year after I had been declared terminal. They found that my heart had returned to normal, the lung was functioning again, and—can you believe it?—my eroded kidney had regenerated itself. There were no traces of the tuberculosis. I was given a clean bill of health."

Another year would pass before she would be able to piece together the puzzle of her recovery. Finally, after having read through a stack of old chemistry textbooks, she concluded that it was the folic acid in the spinach that had brought about her recovery.

"We were in the Dark Ages of health in those days," she said, shaking her head. "There was nothing to read, really, and no one to talk to about nutrition. I was on my own. Out of necessity, to keep myself well, I began to study the chemistry of foods."

A week after our second visit I went up to Sapello again.

I found Dr. Parcells in the sunporch of her home visiting with three German doctors. The conversation was highly technical: healing with magnetic currents, with color, with sound vibrations. At one point during the meeting she took a phone call from a former student whose mother was suffering the first onslaught of Alzheimer's disease.

"Sounds like a lack of oxygen to the brain, Honey," Dr. Parcells said into the receiver. "Is she cleaning her food? Well, do it *for* her."

It had been a busy week. She had been on the phone recommending nutritional plans to two other borderline Alzheimer's clients, a young man recently diagnosed as HIV-positive, a woman who was beginning to experience paralysis in the lower half of her body (Dr. Parcells immediately asked her whether she had undergone a hysterectomy—she had), a man with prostate cancer (she asked him whether he had been around X rays and was told that, since he was a dentist, he was around X rays all the time), a young woman with a disfiguring skin problem, and a former employee who, inexplicably, had been losing weight and feeling fatigued (she told him it sounded like parasites). She had also received two visits a day from people wanting advice and had entertained one "elderly" couple who had no physical complaints but had heard about her and flown out from New York simply to spend a few hours with her.

The doctors left, and she and I sat down to dinner. "Once I understood how I had regained my health, I started learning the age-old principles of nature. The body has its own healing mechanism. If it isn't clogged up with toxins, it will perform beautifully on its own. The body is wise—much wiser than we give it credit for being."

Our meal was plain, but delicious—roasted chicken, brown rice, a green salad, and a dish of steamed carrots and broccoli. Later I would be able to recognize the meal's deceptively simple food combinations, calculated according to Dr. Parcells's research in food chemistry for optimum digestion and nourishment: one protein, one whole-grain (non-gluten-based) starch, and three vegetables, two of which grew above ground and one that grew below ground. Everything we were eating had been cleaned before cooking in a water-and-bleach solution.

"I became a teacher out of necessity," she said. "I wanted to stay healthy, so I studied whatever was available. Gradually I began to share information with my friends, and they had good results applying it to their own health problems. Eventually I was asked to speak to small groups, then larger groups. You know, people are smart: they can take a little good information and help themselves."

She moved to Texas, then to southern California, where, in 1950, she was asked to set up a school of nutrition at Sierra States University, an advanced naturopathic college dedicated to researching and teaching the latest alternative approaches to health.

"At last, I was in my element. During the day I had a full schedule of classes in a teaching kitchen I designed myself; at night I studied all the new healing theories, including electromagnetic modes of treatment, radiesthesia, and my favorite, color therapy."

My visits to Sapello became more frequent. Twice, sometimes three times a week, I got into my car with notebooks, a tape recorder, and a laptop computer and headed north. Dr. Parcells looked forward to our meetings. She would greet me with her infectious laugh and say, "Well, here's the writer! What are we going to talk about today?"

We talked about whatever was on her mind at the moment. She was particularly interested in what she termed "the feminine energy" coming upon the planet. "Everything will change soon, you see. We've been living in male-dominated ages, and there have been wars and terrible upheavals. Now we're about to get back in touch with 'the mother principle.' In matters of health, we were eager to give up our bodies to other people—like taking our cars in to garage mechanics to be fixed. But soon we'll come to understand that we can care for ourselves and correct our own imbalances."

She spoke about the vital importance of detoxification in a health regime, the proper combination of foods, and the necessity of cleaning foods. She described her original herbal remedies and explained how they worked.

The mention of the word "drugs" would take her off into a diatribe. "Drugs can do terrible harm to the body," she said. "They're either stimulants or depressants. They mask symptoms, which are the only indications we have that something might be out of balance inside. But even if there weren't all these drugs to contend with, we're living in an environment depressed by the overuse of artificial fertilizers and pesticides. Do you realize that everything we eat—everything!—has been grown in a soup of polluted air, lifeless water, and depleted soil?"

I was starting to see the many sides of her personality. On some days she was the benevolent teacher, on other days the scolding prophet. Sometimes she was the soul of patience; at other times she treated me like a lazy student who hadn't done his homework—she would push ahead with a sense of urgency, skip over areas she assumed I already knew, and forge into unfamiliar territory. On those occasions when I would try to bring her back to material I hadn't grasped completely, she would take a deep breath and say, "Look it up—you'll see I'm right."

I was in a graduate class of one.

Two months into our visits it seemed inevitable that I should write a book about Dr. Parcells and her philosophy of natural self-healing. When I suggested it, though, she resisted. The world wasn't ready to hear what she had to say, she told me. Medical authorities would misconstrue her message. They would scoff at her ideas and scorn the value of her research.

I reminded her that a little good information could save lives, as it had saved her life so long ago. But I was trying to persuade into the spotlight someone who had stayed safely in the background for half a century, quietly advocating, but wary of going public to speak for, self-healing.

Back in Santa Fe, I had resigned myself to believing that the rare and wonderful wisdom of Hazel Parcells would die with her, when I received a phone call from her on a snowy afternoon in December.

"I was talking with my spirit guides last night," she said. "It seems I'm supposed to get this information out to as many people as possible. And you're supposed to help me." The next morning I was on the road to Sapello, this time my car loaded down not only with notebooks, the tape recorder, and the computer, but also with my hastily packed suitcase.

I moved into a vacant room in her large ranchhouse, and Dr. Parcells and I spent the next five months plowing through a lifetime's accumulation of papers, books, charts, letters, notes, photographs, and tapes.

Now, as I sifted and sorted through her extensive collection, I began piecing together the details of her own life as a teacher and healer. In 1960, when Sierra States University closed its doors in downtown Los Angeles, a victim of smog, urban decay, and dwindling funding, she embarked on her own practice as a nutritional counselor.

Well into her sixties she garnered a sheaf of diplomas: Doctor of Naturopathy, Doctor of Chiropractic, Doctor of Philosophy in Nutrition.

She had become adept at the esoteric art of radiesthesia and was able to test her clients by consulting a pendulum, which she held over a sample of a person's blood or sputum. In this way she detected imbalances and deficiencies and was able to help people correct them by recommending natural remedies. If she found someone with muscle cramps was lacking calcium, for instance, she consulted her radiesthesia board to learn if adding calcium to the diet would end the condition. If the results were positive, she suggested use of the supplement. It was a simple and entirely noninvasive procedure, but the results were remarkably effective. People spoke of "miracle cures," but Dr. Parcells dismissed those claims: "Only taxidermists and undertakers do *curing*," she said. "And as for miracles, no, it's just nature's way."

At the age of seventy-five, she opened a second office in Albuquerque and commuted monthly across the Arizona desert in her car to keep appointments. A few years later, fleeing the big-city environmental problems of southern California, she made a permanent move to New Mexico, where she continued to advise clients and teach classes.

All her groundbreaking work during that time was meticulously documented, but the documentation was everywhere—in boxes, folders, and file cabinets, on shelves, and in large stacks on tables and desktops in the several rooms of her house. At first, the task of organizing all her research appeared daunting, almost overwhelming. But as we worked through it, a few signposts arose: cleansing programs, the nutrient quality of foods, the proper food combinations for optimum digestion, health in the home, the essentials of her "kitchen chemistry," nature's self-correcting mechanisms.

We worked together at the computer for about six hours a day. When I needed a break, I would excuse myself, rub my eyes, and go outside for a few gulps of mountain air. She stayed behind at our desk and, by the time I returned, was ready with more facts and new approaches to the material. Her stamina, fueled by a sense of urgency to dispatch her message to the world, was amazing.

Slowly, the many hundreds of separate pieces of information she had amassed over sixty-five years laboring in the vineyards of human health began to attach themselves to seven simple and practical steps to total wellness—the Seven Steps of the Parcells Method.

In the late spring I returned home to Santa Fe and continued reworking the material for this book. Every two weeks or so I went back up to Sapello to check the accuracy of information with Dr. Parcells and add fine points to the nearly completed manuscript. I would ask her if she were in the mood to work, and she would say, "You bet I am!" Dr. Parcells loved work and felt a visit was not complete unless some "useful" information passed between us.

When she celebrated her 106th birthday in September, I brought her a big bouquet of wildflowers. She donned an old-fashioned bonnet and a pair of oversized sunglasses, and we sat on her front porch; we must have looked like two jaded tourists off on a cruise.

"Now that the book is finished, I think all the loose ends are tied up," she said. "Let's hope it's a good seed we've planted."

She took the wildflowers in her hands and inhaled deeply. "Have I ever told you this story? When I was girl of about seven or eight, I had been invited to a birthday party at a neighboring farm. My father picked a bouquet of chrysanthemums for me to give to the birthday girl. I was awfully disappointed, because I knew the other children would be bringing store-bought toys and such. But when I presented my flowers at the party, everybody loved them. They were the talk of the party. Nature's gifts are always the best, don't you agree?"

She was quiet for a moment, then her face opened in her familiar smile and she turned to me. "It must be a hundred years since my father gave me those chrysanthemums, and, you know, I can still see them and smell their fragrance."

Four months later Dr. Parcells passed away peacefully in her sleep. Her gift to us is the information in this book, which she saw as a way for all of us to grasp the reins of our own lives, to bring ourselves back to a place of caring for our own health, and to take responsibility for the wellness of our bodies. With a little good information, she believed, we all can live happy, healthy lives to one hundred and beyond.

Its message is that we have the power within us to enjoy our birthright of physical well-being, if we call upon nature's sublime principles and use them to help us on the road to total and lasting health.

It is a message of hope.

DECIDING TO BE HEALTHY

This is not an easy time to be healthy. Everything in our experience pulls us in the other direction, away from health. Manufactured foods available to us are empty of the necessary nutrients for life; our drinking water is lifeless, lacking precious minerals; the air we breathe is poisoned. Attempting to remain in health in this kind of situation calls for character—for perseverance, fortitude, and ingenuity.

Still, there are a lot of things we *can* do to create wellness for ourselves and to live the picture of health.

Most of us lead busy lives. Usually we don't give a second thought to our physical condition unless something begins to break down in us. We may suffer some nagging, but mild, discomfort—heartburn, gas, decreased energy, muscle aches, constipation—but we treat these symptoms with drugs, either under the care of a health professional or, more likely, on our own. We are relatively healthy.

If our health problems become worse, we go for help and receive it in the form of well-intentioned advice, which is often attached to things to take for our ailments. We begin to feel better, and for the moment we *are* better. So often, though, the underlying cause of our initial trouble is never plumbed. When we begin to slide back into ill health, we reach out again for what helped us in the past and, once again, obtain some relief. Meanwhile, the real problem lies hidden under the stimulants and depressants we used merely to end our discomfort. And now the drugs we took to shut off our symptoms have added to our problems, building up in the body to form a virtual toxic dump.

Dr. Hazel Parcells understood that our bodies have their own natural ways of staying healthy—*but only under the condition that we allow nature the opportunity to operate in us.* That will happen when we stop taking toxins into our bodies, clean out the toxins that have accumulated there, and let nature take its healing course.

Once we are rid of the poisons that are plaguing us, we can begin to build lasting health. In our world, that's not as easy as it may sound. We are living in a wash of environmental toxins. Over the span of a century, our planet's natural life-sustaining capabilities have been compromised by the wide and indiscriminate use of all kinds of toxic substances. To live in health today calls for diligence and dedication, but the rewards of staying healthy are enormous; they are nothing less than joy, peace of mind, a constant sense of delight, and the fullness of life.

This book is for everyone who is deciding to reclaim the birthright of lasting health. It is a how-to manual for all of us— from the half-healthy to the chronically ill—who are reaching for wellness by turning to nature's way.

All the information here is simple and practical. All of it is aimed at developing in us the joyful state of physical well-being. Anyone can follow these seven steps to better health and discover what "miracles" of well-being await right around the corner. There are no easy fixes, however. Dr. Parcells used to say, "If you want to be healthy, you have to trade your wishbone for a backbone and get to work!" The Seven Step Program of the Parcells Method calls us to find that backbone of determination in ourselves, to roll up our sleeves, and begin working at our own health. But building true health, you will find, is also a joyful and deeply satisfying experience.

All the recommendations in this book can be taken up right where you are right now—whether you are young, middle-aged, or elderly; whether you are enjoying good health most of the time or are caught in the grip of a chronic illness. If you are sincerely interested in enhancing the quality of your life, you can start today to increase your life-energy, to build up your immune system, to walk the path of exhilarating well-being.

Let this book help you as you begin your miraculous journey.

Live Better Longer

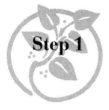

Step 1

CLEAN BODY INSIDE

*If we put fresh, new wine into an old wineskin, the new wine
will turn sour and be worthless. The same principle is at work
in matters of health. A healthy body begins with cleaning out
the accumulated toxins of the past and preparing it to accept
new and effective nutrients. When the body is cleared of poisons, nature will take over and provide us the gift of health.*

DR. HAZEL PARCELLS

HALF-HEALTHY

In spite of all the diet and health programs that have been put
forth over the years, we still are a nation of unhealthy people.
A full third of us are clinically obese; the statistics on cancer, heart
disease, and other tragic diseases mount each year; degenerative disorders like rheumatoid arthritis, osteoporosis, diabetes, hypertension, and ulcerative colitis continue on the increase, even with the
miraculous advances in technology we've achieved.

Dr. Hazel Parcells observed that most people are not terribly ill most of the time. Most people don't suffer from the ravages of a physical disorder that plagues them continually and controls their lives. But over the years she began to see indications that, while most people are not ill most of the time, they are not healthy all the time, either. She called this condition "half-healthy": not entirely ill, but not entirely well.

A half-healthy person is able to get up in the morning and go to work or engage in some other form of activity. The person drags through the day, tires out, and crawls into bed at night. The overriding theme of the day is exhaustion; smaller subthemes relate to little aches and pains, headaches, stomach troubles, digestive problems, unclear thinking, insomnia, and low energy.

The half-healthy person is rarely ever totally enthusiastic, cheerful, relaxed, or happy. Something is always tugging at the sleeve. The problem may be minor as physical ailments go, but something's there, and it's worrisome.

Symptoms of the half-healthy find their expression on the shelves of pharmacies, supermarkets, and wherever else drugs or druglike substances are sold over the counter, including the aisles of health food stores. Television commercials and slick magazine ads deliver illustrated catalogues of half-healthy ills: nausea, indigestion, gas, sleeplessness, lack of concentration, diarrhea, skin irritations, fatigue, constipation, irritability, cramps, anxiety, depression, and all the rest. We spend increasing billions of dollars on health care every year—not only on traditional medical care, but also on alternative and self-help health approaches. Still, true and lasting health continues to elude us.

The peculiar thing about our predicament is that never before in history have we had a better opportunity to be well all the time.

More information comes our way daily, even hourly, via television and radio, the computer, and magazines and newspapers to increase our knowledge about how to take care of ourselves. More tools are available today, and more practitioners trained to use them. We *should* be more healthy now than ever before.

Number of U.S. Deaths from Cancer

1937	144,774	
1960	330,700	228 % increase
1987	476,700	303 % increase

(Source: U.S. Bureau of the Census)

U.S. Death Rates from Cancer 1970–1990 (per 100,000 persons)

	Male	Female
1970	182.1	144.4
1980	205.3	163.6
1990	221.3	186.0

(Source: U.S. Bureau of the Census)

U.S. Expenditures on Health Care (per person)

1929	$29.49
1940	29.62
1955	105.38
1970	343.44
1993	3,299.00

(Source: U.S. Health Care Financing Administration)

OUR WORLD A CENTURY AGO

In 1889, when Dr. Parcells was born, our world was quite a different place. It was predominantly an agrarian world in which most people grew virtually all their own food and ate it fresh from the unspoiled fields that surrounded their homes.

Crops were plentiful, and they were permeated with high-quality, life-enhancing nutrients from nature. Food was most often eaten when it was harvested; for out-of-season eating, it was preserved by natural methods such as drying, smoking, and cooling.

The water that brought foods to life was clear, clean, and full of energy. The air in which foods thrived was pure and sweet. The soil that nurtured them was rich with natural minerals, alive, and in perfect balance.

"Pests" were kept away from the food supply by natural means, using home remedies, or simply growing crops in rotation or planting certain crops near or away from other crops.

On the family farm in 1889, enough was grown so the members of the family could eat well and perhaps have a bit left over to share with others. Farm animals helped in the growing of food and enjoyed the fruits of their toil along with their human caretakers.

Farm people lived close to the earth. They understood the movements of the seasons and prepared and provided for them. They also knew the seasons of their own lives—the meaning of birth, of death, and of all the rich and beautiful times in between.

A powerful life force was upon the planet, and all who lived on it and from it possessed the benefits of nature in its energetic fullness.

Percentage of the U.S. Population in Farm Occupations

1850	63.7	1950	11.6
1870	53.0	1960	6.1
1900	37.5	1970	3.6
1920	27.0	1980	2.7
1930	21.2	1990	2.4
1940	17.4		

(Source: Economic Research Service, U.S. Department of Agriculture)

Number and Size of Farms 1940–1992

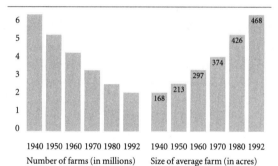

1940 1950 1960 1970 1980 1992   1940 1950 1960 1970 1980 1992
Number of farms (in millions)   Size of average farm (in acres)

(Source: U.S. Department of Agriculture)

"PROGRESS"

The year Dr. Parcells was born, a margarine factory employee in New York testified to a state investigator that his work making margarine made his hands so sore that his nails came loose, his hair dropped out, and he had to be confined to

Bellevue Hospital for general debility. The butter substitute, which was marketed as "pure creamery butter," was actually manufactured from hog fat and bleaches.

Modern commercial techniques were entering the realm of our food supply as Dr. Parcells was entering the world. During her childhood, society was still free of the devastating effects of big business on natural food, but all of that would change rapidly in the first few decades of the twentieth century.

A hundred years ago a great appetite for "progress" filled the national consciousness and, as the population grew, that appetite grew. The greatest growth in all sectors of society centered around how to meet the appetite for expansion in the area of "progress."

In time, our needs became greater by far than anything we had to deal with in the past. No one could have known, as we embarked on this path of unqualified "progress," how enormous our growing demands would be. Before we had fully understood what was taking place, our needs had increased beyond our ability to fulfill them.

Total Assets from Farming 1940–1970
(in billions of dollars)

Year	Assets
1940	52.9
1945	94.2
1950	132.5
1955	165.1
1960	203.5
1965	237.2
1970	305.8

(Source: U.S. Department of Agriculture)

In the United States each year, over 1.2 billion pounds of pesticides and herbicides are sprayed or added to crops. That amounts to roughly 10 pounds of pesticides for each man, woman, and child. Although the pesticides are designed to combat insects and other organisms, experts estimate that only 2 percent of the pesticide actually serves its purpose, while over 98 percent of the pesticide is absorbed into the air, water, soil, or food supply. Most pesticides in use are synthetic chemicals of questionable safety. Major long-term health risks of these include increased likelihood of cancer and birth defects; major health risks of acute intoxication include vomiting, diarrhea, blurred vision, tremors, convulsions, and nerve damage.

Michael T. Murray, N.D., in *The Healing Power of Foods*, 1993

FOOD AND MONEY

When science, driven by commerce, undertook to stimulate our food supply for greater production, it couldn't have known what was going to happen. Predicting the outcome of a global chemical chain reaction begun with simple soil "enhancement" or the elimination of a few garden pests would have been impossible a century ago. Even if we could have known the possible consequences, moneymaking considerations would probably have overridden them. Our attitudes about food were beginning to change. Gradually, food moved from being a source of life to a source of profit.

Food meant money: if more food could be grown, more money could be made. To grow more food required "management" of nature, much as one would manage any other industrial resource.

Pesticides and commercial fertilizers were introduced. Suddenly, the soil of earth was becoming a large outdoor factory. Big agriculture, using industrial methods of production, managed the food supply—applying artificial chemicals to food in the fields to prolong shelf life and dressing crops with a cosmetic shine to make them appear eternally "in season."

OUR WORLD NOW

Now we're left with the terrible legacy of our lack of awareness. We went out, science in hand, to develop a certain vision, but without understanding all the laws of nature. We raided and plundered some areas of the natural realm to overstimulate and overgrow other areas. In the process, we upset nature's balance.

Today, as a result, much of our water is contaminated and sour; the air of our cities and farms alike is foul and thick with invisible toxins; our soil is largely without growing energy, pathetically exhausted, incapable of fostering and sustaining life.

The "food" from these polluted sources does not nourish us. In fact, it does just the opposite—it depresses and diminishes the life force in us and erodes our ability to withstand the attacks of organisms foreign to our bodies. As our environment weakens, our bodies become vulnerable to the unnatural conditions brought on by an altered ecosystem. Lack of true nourishment results in depressed immunity, opening the door to ever increasing epidemics of physical disorders in all areas of planetary life.

We're living longer today, but, ironically, we may be in ill health much of the time. A staggering statistic: annual health expenditures in the United States alone now total more than $884 billion.

Health Effects of Common Pesticides

Name	Class	Major Crop Use	Health Effects
Captan	Fungicide	Apples, peaches, almonds, seeds	Probable human carcinogen; mutagen; causes reproductive effects in animals; possible teratogen.
Daminozide	Growth regulator	Apples, peanuts	Probable human carcinogen; causes multiple tumors at many sites in animals including the lungs, liver, pancreas, nasal tissue, and vascular system; mutagen.
Mancozeb	Fungicide	Apples, onions, potatoes, tomatoes, small grains	Probable human carcinogen; mutagen; causes birth defects in experimental animals; affects kidney, thyroid, and prostrate glands.
Mevinphos	Insecticide	Many fruits and vegetables	Affects nervous system; possible mutagen.
Parathion	Insecticide	Citrus, cotton, orchard crops, vegetables, fruits	Possible human carcinogen; mutagen; extremely toxic; causes nervous system effects; affects eyes in animals.
Quintozene	Fungicide	Vegetables, small grains	Probable human carcinogen; causes liver tumors in animals; possible developmental effects.

(Source: Environmental Protection Agency)

A CLOSER LOOK: CHEMICALS

In the early part of this century manufactured chemicals began to be applied to food. These applications were in three major areas: the expansion of food production, the destruction of grasses and insects, and the management of food for preservation.

The entire effort was pursued as a commercial enterprise. Destroying grasses, weeds, and insects would allow crops a better yield and therefore make them more economical to produce. The destruction of pests was extended from crops to livestock, which, though on an entirely different scale of natural life, were treated as if they were carrots or corn: in the same way crops were sprayed with insecticides to protect them from pests, animals were shot with chemical antibiotics to protect them from disease.

Pushing growth into overabundance seemed to be the key concept. But the only way to reach that unnatural goal was to kill off part of life, and the killing was done with manufactured chemicals—poisons.

THE ARTIFICIAL MANAGEMENT OF FOOD AND OUR HEALTH

Unless we're growing our own food in our own backyards, we're eating food supplied to us by artificial laws of growth and expansion, which are contrary to the laws of nature.

Isn't it logical to suppose that foods manipulated by *artificial* means from the field to the grocery store are going to provide *artificial* support to the body—which is to say no support at all, since our bodies can use only natural sustenance?

All the elements that have been put into our food chain—to gain higher crop yields, to kill bugs, to kill weeds, and so on—reduce the natural life force in foods down to their own poisonous level.

Food carries the energy of the soil it is grown in. If soil has been modified, depleted, and manipulated, the results will appear in our food. Low-energy food, consequently, will take its toll on our bodies. It's not difficult to trace the cause of so much illness and so many degenerative disorders. The breakdown of our soils and the deterioration of our health are intrinsically related.

> *Artificial manures lead inevitably to artificial nutrition, artificial food, artificial animals, and finally, to artificial men and women.*
>
> Dr. Bernard Jensen and Mark Anderson, in *Empty Harvest*, 1990

WHAT WE CAN DO

After a long lifetime spent observing human health, Dr. Parcells came to believe that virtually all health problems are the result of malnutrition. If we were nourished properly, she thought, we would suffer far fewer illnesses than we do—perhaps none at all.

She also believed, by the same token, that most physical disorders have environmental origins. This is not to discount the effects of factors like genetics or circumstances at birth. Neither does it dismiss what we ourselves do to compromise our own health. However, she firmly supported the premise that a depressed environment was directly responsible for most illnesses—not only in the human world, but in the animal and plant kingdoms as well.

In that conclusion she saw a great deal to be distressed about—but she also saw a ray of hope. As long as we are aware that our environment is not conducive to our health, then we can actually do something to change our situation. We can begin to restore the environment to its natural state. And, meanwhile, we can protect ourselves from our polluted surroundings, making our own personal environment work *for* our health, rather than against it.

Immunity from illness can only come by way of food. The only way to build health is to put good, clean food and water into bodies that have been cleared of toxins. Nature will do the rest.

MY OWN EXPERIENCE

When I met Dr. Hazel Parcells I was a reasonably healthy fifty-year-old man who watched what I ate, exercised vigorously three times a week, and in general took care of myself. I used food supplements off and on. I had given up smoking cigarettes a few years before (it had been very difficult, and I lapsed back a few times). Every couple of months, to "tune up," I went to an acupuncturist for a treatment. I rarely suffered any illness more than an annoying cold, and when one came, it didn't last long. I had been hospitalized only once in my life, when I was nine, to have my tonsils out.

Still, I was twenty-five pounds overweight—something I just couldn't shake all my adult life (I had been an overweight child). My blood pressure hovered in the "borderline-high" area. I used antacid mints a few times a week and a stronger antacid liquid if my stomach got really irritated. I drank a lot of coffee, took aspirins to calm down, and used sleeping pills to get to sleep at night. My energy level was just so-so; if I could fit in an afternoon nap, I would.

And something else: in the past two years I noticed that my skin had begun to turn progressively darker.

In short, I was one of the "half-healthy."

Cleaning House

Dr. Parcells put me on a detoxification and rejuvenation program that lasted eight days, and amazing things began to happen.

First, my skin cleared up, from a dark brown to a healthy glowing pink—at the end of the eight days my skin actually looked like the skin of a baby. My weight became manageable: I lost twelve pounds doing the weeklong program. I gained back four pounds in the week after I was finished with the program, stabilized for a month, then began to lose an average of two pounds a month after that until I reached my proper weight.

My energy soared. My blood pressure measured normal. I found I could work for several hours at a stretch without wanting to take a nap and get through the day and night with no help from drugs of any kind—including those I had considered rather harmless ones like caffeine, indigestion candies, laxatives, and aspirins.

I also had a new outlook on life. I felt revived, eager for challenges, ready to start off in new directions. I felt that whole worlds of possibilities were waiting for me—doors that had been closed were swung wide open. A kind of expansion of spirit came over me.

What I had experienced was not only a physical cleansing, but also a deep emotional, psychological, and spiritual cleansing.

I had never felt better in my life. The cleansing program Dr. Parcells recommended for me literally "cleaned house," as she said, and allowed my body to take over the work of healing itself—naturally, easily, and effectively.

In my case, the liver was congested and clogged with poisons, to the point where it wasn't able to do its best work of processing and purifying. The blocked-up liver had caused a slowdown of my ability to burn food, especially fat, thus keeping me overweight. Its decreased function also had caused accumulations of unassimilated foods, food supplements, and medicines to putrefy in me, further bogging down the liver's activity; the result was that a variety of aches and pains were surfacing from a number of places, my sleep was being hindered, and my skin had darkened to a complexion that looked turbid, congested, and unhealthy.

"If you take your foot off the brake, your car will go faster," Dr. Parcells said to me when we went over the results of my eight-day adventure. It was a lesson I learned by doing, and the outcome was more positive than I could have imagined.

DETOXIFICATION AND REJUVENATION AT THE CELL LEVEL

Dr. Parcells developed her cleansing program in the 1950s and 1960s. She recommended it to people who came to her sincerely wanting to turn their health around. It was always the first step for all her health-building plans.

The Parcells Detoxification and Rejuvenation Program works at the cell level. It is not a simple stomach evacuation or bowel cleanse. It is not a mere rest-from-food regime for the internal organs. It actually loosens and removes toxic wastes that have been stored in the body for years.

This program works on many levels to clean the whole person. Its impact on the physical level is the most obvious and the most dramatic, of course, but it also clears blockages on the emotional level (or the emotional body, as some are calling it) and affects many other aspects of a person's life, including one's psychological and spiritual sides. If anger and resentment have been stored in the body for many years, they are given the opportunity of leaving at this time. If some self-destructive psychological patterns have gotten stuck in the mind and have spilled over into the body, they can dissolve during this program.

Complete directions for the Parcells Detoxification and Rejuvenation Program are given in Appendix I, at the back of the book.

OTHER DETOXIFICATION PROGRAMS

You will find other detoxification and rejuvenation programs at your local health food store or from herbal specialists and naturopathic or holistic practitioners. New health food supermarkets stock many fine products that perform well. Some are short, one- or two-day regimes. Others, like the famous Master Fast (lemon juice, maple syrup, and cayenne pepper) can be longer in duration.

Any one of these detoxification programs will clean the body on the inside. For help in deciding which program to follow, consult your health care professional.

A reminder: during any detoxification and rejuvenation program, one or two colonics, which clear the lower intestine of debris, can be enormously helpful.

For general detoxification, short of cleansing at the cell level, Dr. Parcells recommended one of these regimes:

• Fruit Day: During an entire day, eat only fruit. Eat until you are satisfied, but not so full that you feel bloated. Good "washing" fruits are melons, especially in season. Citrus fruits are also good, with grapefruit heading the list. Eat fruit separately:

an apple or two, then later strawberries, and so on. Drink plenty of water. A Fruit Day can be done as often as once a week.

- Fruit Weekend: For two full consecutive days, eat only fruit, as described above.

- Vegetable Juice Day: Juice fresh vegetables (preferably in season) and sip on the juice through the day. Remember to drink at least eight 8-ounce glasses of water throughout the day.

- Apple Juice and Chlorophyll Day: Drink 8 ounces of organic apple juice mixed with 1 teaspoon of liquid chlorophyll three times through the day. Drink plain apple juice mixed with an equal amount of water as hunger dictates. Drink plenty of water.

- Rest-from-Food Day: Eat no food at all for one day. Drink plenty of liquids, including herbals teas, vegetable broth, and water.

Note: It is vitally important to work *into* a fast and to work *out of* it. On the day before an All-Fruit Day, for instance, cut your food intake back to about half of a normal day's eating—and especially go lightly on the evening meal or skip it entirely. On the day after the fast, do the same in reverse: eat lightly (begin with fruits and vegetables, then introduce proteins, then, last of all, complex carbohydrates like bread and pasta).

Break a fast gradually and with awareness. The best way is to choose an easily digestible fresh fruit or vegetable and chew it slowly, feeling the effects of the food's power to feed the body and bring about health.

If you commit to a fast, do it. Cravings may come up, but to abruptly end a fast with a candy bar or a slice of pizza can do harm to the system. It's best to calmly decide to do without food, go through with it to the end you set at the start, and reintroduce food slowly until you are back to normal eating patterns.

To correct feelings associated with low blood sugar—lightheadedness or a "fading" feeling—mix half a teaspoon of salt in warm water and sip on it.

It always helps to tell people close to you what you are doing when starting a cleansing program and to ask for their support.

THERAPEUTIC BATHING

Therapeutic baths help the body throw off accumulated toxins through the skin, the largest eliminative organ of the body, enhancing the cleansing process.

Use any one or more of the four Parcells Therapeutic Baths listed in Step Two as part of your detoxification and rejuvenation program. Therapeutic bathing should be done in the evening before retiring, only one bath per evening. Follow the directions to the letter.

BENEFITS OF A DETOXIFICATION PROGRAM

What a detoxification and rejuvenation program will do for you:

• Carry off toxic debris that has been stored away and building up in your body.

• End or mitigate all "half-healthy" symptoms such as indigestion, bloating, headaches, food allergies, fatigue, migraines, most hypertension, and other aches, pains, and complaints associated with the results of poor eating habits.

Recommended Reading on Other Detoxification
and Rejuvenation Programs

Bragg, Paul, C. *The Miracle of Fasting.* Desert Hot Springs,
CA: Health Science, 1976.

Ehret, Arnold. *Rational Fasting for Physical, Mental
and Spiritual Rejuvenation.* Beaumont, CA: Ehret
Literature, 1971.

Kellog, J. H. *The New Dietetics.* Battle Creek, MI: Modern
Medicine, 1927.

Lindlahr, Henry. *Natural Cure.* Poona, India: Dr. M. B.
Godbole, 1937.

Macfadden, B. *Fasting for Health.* New York: Macfadden,
1924.

McCoy, F. *The Fast Way to Health.* Los Angeles:
McCoy, 1926.

Cited in Christopher Hobbs, *Foundations of Health,* 1992,
an excellent guide to self-healing with herbs and foods in
general and detoxification in particular.

• Speed up your metabolism as your body's internal organs kick
  into gear casting off poisons (by the way, if a detoxification
  program is done properly, most people feel very little or no
  hunger for food on it).

• Prepare your body to accept true nourishment from clean
  food and clean water.

• Purge your emotional body of old, toxic feelings.

- Allow you to see old psychological patterns and release them if you find they don't work for you now.

- Open your mind and heart to new emotional, psychological, and spiritual sustenance.

What you need to do to prepare for a detoxification and rejuvenation program:

- See your health care professional and ask if there would be anything in the program that might be harmful to you. Because you are doing a cleaning, no drugs or food supplements should be taken during the program.

- Find a block of time for yourself—one day, a weekend, or several days for the program and two or three days after that to begin rebuilding health—so you can undertake the program without interruption and with the least amount of disturbance or energy drain (most people find it best not to work during this time). Give yourself a "health vacation." You'll return to "normal" life soon enough, but as a new person with a refreshed body and new attitudes.

- Resolve to take nothing into your body except what is specified by the program—and that includes all drugs, pills, powders, supplements, tobacco, alcohol, sugar, and so on.

- Gather together all the materials you will need to do your program. Don't wait for the first day of the program to do your shopping or you'll sabotage the program—and yourself.

- Tell the people in your life that you are embarking on a health-giving adventure that will enhance your health and ask for their support.

THE PARASITE PROBLEM

When she was teaching at Sierra States University in the 1950s, Dr. Parcells ran an experiment to learn the fate of animal tissue as its environment changed in the absence of oxygen. She took an ordinary uncooked beef roast, put it in an airtight glass container, and observed what happened as it degenerated through several stages of alkalinity to the final end of any evidence of life.

As the animal flesh deteriorated, entering new environments of degeneration, microorganisms appeared in the tissue. Those life forms disappeared as the decline continued, and other vermin made their appearance.

Our physical environment is not unlike the environment of the roast. When it becomes depressed enough in supporting the function of the life force, various forms of pestilence begin to show themselves. Many plagues can materialize or be attracted to us in the weakened state caused by a suppressed life-giving operation in the environment. Among those plagues are parasites.

Parasites are in most of us, but in an inactive form. As long as our immunity (the life-energy of our internal environment) is high, they will not manifest themselves to do their damage. When our immunity is lowered, they will begin to become active.

A doctor from Dallas once came to see me. He was a horrible sight, his body covered all over with red sores. He had contracted a vicious, parasitic worm while in India and had lived with the problem for two years. Nothing he prescribed for himself and nothing prescribed for him by others helped.

> When he walked into my office he said, "Look here, if you can't help me, I'm ready to end it all."
>
> It was a tough case of parasites, and it took three months of hard work to clear up. After the doctor completed a nutritional program I formulated for him to rid his system of the problem and built himself up with the proper food, he was fine. He has since referred many other people, including other doctors, to me for help with similar problems.
>
> Dr. Hazel Parcells

The Prevalence of Parasites

Americans today are host to more than 130 different kinds of parasites ranging from microscopic organisms to foot-long tapeworms. Practically every imaginable kind of exotic parasitic disorder has been found on our shores: African sleeping sickness, toxoplasmosis, schistosomiasis, giardiasis, amebiasis, filariasis, even malaria. Although parasites are an insidious health threat, most people in the United States are unaware of their pervasive presence, because they think such problems occur only in developing countries.

Many seemingly unrelated factors unique to our modern lifestyles have contributed to an unrestrained parasite epidemic. Some of these factors include the rise in international travel, the contamination of municipal and rural water supplies, the increasing use of day-care centers, the influx of refugee and immigrant populations from endemic areas, the indiscriminate use of antibiotics and immunosuppressive drugs, and the sexual revolution.

The problem is so acute that some sources claim as much as 25 percent of the population of metropolitan New York may be infected. Projections for the year 2025 suggest that more than half of the 8.3 billion people on earth then will have parasitic conditions. Other reports and predictions are even more ominous. One recent study suggests that as many as 80 percent of the world's people are now infected with parasites.

Indications that a person may have parasites (these are the most common indications, but the presence of one or more of them could also signal a different health problem) include:

Drowsiness after eating

Anemia

Constipation

Allergies

Bloating and gas

Unclear thinking

"Toxic" feeling

Explosive diarrhea

Ulcers

Tendency for blood clots

Jaundice

High or low blood-sugar levels

Mineral imbalance

Fluid buildup during full moon

Light-colored, fatty stools

Recurrent yeast infections

Joint pain

Asthma

Grinding of teeth during sleep

Liver problems

Malnutrition

All Worms Are Parasites, but Not All Parasites Are Worms

A parasite is a very small life form that can be either an irritant or a destroyer or both. The ones that cannot live in the presence of oxygen are commonly found in the intestinal tract, a place containing very little oxygen, where they are nourished and propagate.

Parasites are responsible for many conditions for which no apparent cause can be found. When Dr. Parcells investigated the health problems of ten people, six of them showed indications of worms or other parasites. While these microbes can be present anywhere in the body, the most common are found in the intestinal tract.

The many different types of parasites each produce their own effect. For example, amoebas, one of the most common of the parasites, interfere with the digestive process; they can disturb digestion in a person for years.

Worms—tapeworms, round stomach worms, and many others—are parasites, but not all parasites are worms. Because many are microscopic, parasites are unlikely to be found by ordinary means. They wreck livers and therefore whole internal systems. They lodge themselves in the soft tissues in many areas of the body. One of the greatest causes of bleeding ulcers is parasites.

When sufferers are rid of the parasites that have been breaking down their bodies, there is a dramatic return to normal health. That does not guarantee there will be no reinfection, however.

Parasites are now a part of living in an environment that has been compromised in its life-nurturing abilities by toxins in the air, the soil, and the water. Our depressed environment opens us to degenerative conditions of many kinds and makes us prey to plagues of parasites that ordinarily would never enter our experience.

When we look at what is keeping the vast majority of people in the world half-healthy, surely we must point to parasites as one of the causes. They themselves are appearing more and more frequently now that there is an environment to support them—an environment, diminished by contamination and mistreatment, that is becoming less competent to sustain human life.

Testing for Parasites

To find out if you have parasites, see your medical doctor or alternative health care professional. There are many ways of testing for parasites: the most common among them is testing a stool sample (this has to be done in a laboratory). Other ways of testing for parasites are kinesiology and dowsing.

Adverse Side Effects of Drugs Used to Treat Parasites

- Iodoquinol (trade name Yodoxin). *Occasional:* rash, acne, slight enlargement of thyroid gland, nausea, diarrhea, cramps, anal pruritus. *Rare:* optic atrophy, loss of vision, peripheral neutropathy after prolonged use in high dosage (months), iodine sensitivity.

- Metronidazole (trade name Flagyl). *Frequent:* nausea, headache, dry mouth, metallic taste. *Occasional:* vomiting, diarrhea, insomnia, weakness, stomatitis, vertigo, aparesthesia, rash, dark urine, urethral burning. *Rare:* seizures, encephalopathy, pseudo-membranous colitis, ataxia, leukopenia, peripheral neuropathy, pancreatitis.

- Quinacrine HCl (trade name Atabrine). *Frequent:* dizziness, headache, vomiting, diarrhea. *Occasional:* yellow staining of skin, toxic psychosis, insomnia, bizarre dreams, blood dyscrasias, urticaria, blue and black nail pigmentation, psoriasis-like rash. *Rare:* acute hepatic necrosis, convulsions, severe exfoliative dermatitis, ocular effects similar to those caused by chloroquine.

Hulda Regehr Clark, Ph.D., N.D., in *The Cure for All Cancers,* 1993

Dr. Parcells's Programs

As early as the 1950s, Dr. Parcells was finding that many health problems attributed to other causes—or considered of unknown origin—actually originated with parasites in the body. She developed two purging programs that have been effective down through the years.

If it is determined that you are carrying parasites and you would like information on these two programs, contact:

Parcells Center
P. O. Box 2129
Santa Fe, NM 87504–2129
1–800–811–6784

WHAT YOU CAN DO TODAY FOR BETTER HEALTH

- Be aware that we are living in a natural environment depressed by industrial wastes, fossil fuel emissions, modern methods of agriculture, and other contaminating side effects of our high-technology culture.

- Understand that a depressed environment has brought on a lack of life-energy in our foods and that, in turn, has resulted in a condition in us that nutrition pioneer Dr. Hazel Parcells called "half-healthy."

- Realize that to be healthy all the time today we need to cleanse our bodies from the inside, so that they can accept true nourishment from clean, high-energy food and water.

- Consider taking responsibility for your own health by cleaning toxins out of your body using the Parcells Detoxification and Rejuvenation Program, which cleanses at the cell level, or one of the other programs that will clear your body and make it receptive to good nourishment.

- Understand that working on your health and reaping the rewards of good health is easy, natural, and, most of all, fun. Health brings joy, and lasting health brings with it the fullness of life.

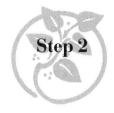

Step 2

CLEAN BODY OUTSIDE

Our bodies need to be clean on the outside as well as on the inside to be truly prepared to receive the life-energy in nutrient-rich food. Through our largest organ, the skin, our bodies collect toxins from daily "wear and tear" in a compromised environment. To free ourselves of pollutants and enhance elimination, I have developed detoxification regimes based on the ancient science of therapeutic bathing. Their effectiveness in restoring health convinces me that they are part of the future of medicine.

DR. HAZEL PARCELLS

IT'S A JUNGLE OUT THERE

Early one winter morning at Sapello I went looking for Dr. Parcells and found her outdoors scooping up a pile of newly fallen snow into a glass pie dish. When I asked her what she was doing, she smiled up at me impishly and asked me to help her bring the snow into her lab.

"We're going to do a little experiment," she said. "I'm curious to see how much radiation is in our air."

I was quite surprised to hear her mention the word "radiation." If any place on earth was free of radiation, surely it must be this isolated, pristine mountain valley hundreds of miles from the nearest urban center.

When we got to the lab and she measured the snow for its radiation content, however, she found levels that one would have expected from living in the shadow of a nuclear weapons plant or an atomic-powered electrical facility. I was amazed—and suddenly began to feel very vulnerable. I asked her if the readings could be correct.

"Oh, yes, they're correct, all right. You see, radiation is airborne. It's everywhere."

That day I began to learn about the dangerous levels of radiation in the air we breathe—and about many other environmental toxins that have become part of daily life. Some of those other environmental dangers to health are X rays, which are another form of radiation and can diminish the effectiveness of the immune system; the irradiation of foods, which extends shelf life but smothers the life-giving, natural nutrients foods are supposed to contain; carbon monoxide, the colorless, odorless gas that robs our air of oxygen; and heavy metals, such as mercury and aluminum.

Nationally and internationally we are making some progress in ridding our environment of these poisons, but we still have a way to go.

Meanwhile, there *are* simple, easy ways to make our personal environment a clean and healthy one.

THERAPEUTIC BATHS

Bathing for health goes back to ancient times. Our distant ancestors used therapeutic bathing as a means of obtaining relief from many bodily disorders. The curative powers of bathing are recorded in the histories of past civilizations alongside the great accomplishments of generals, statesmen, and kings.

Four thousand years ago, the Egyptians developed bathing into a high art, using exotic mineral salts and precious scented oils to spice their water therapies. Greeks of the classical period institutionalized it, housing public baths in grand edifices designed after temples. Ancient Romans took bathing another step, including it as an integral part of civic life; matters of war and peace were decided while politicians soaked—fortunes, alliances, and reputations were made and ruined in the baths.

In her research into natural self-healing, Dr. Parcells found that therapeutic bathing was an excellent way to foster healthy living in a compromised environment. Her various water therapies were developed over more than half a century of observation and application, with remarkable, positive results. Together with a program of good nutrition, they stand as proven methods to help the body regain and remain in good health.

Therapeutic bathing is another way of cleansing, and therefore of healing. Our skin is an organ of our bodies—the largest organ. Sixty-five percent of body cleansing is accomplished through our skin. Cleaning the skin is a science, from which Dr. Parcells drew four safe and effective—and all-natural—procedures.

- The first rids the body of pesticides and other dangerous chemicals in the environment.

- The second cleans the body (through the skin) of radiation.

- The third works to purify the body of carbon monoxide and heavy metals.

- The fourth is an all-purpose skin acidifier, cleanser, and muscle relaxer.

The Underlying Scientific Principle

The Parcells therapeutic baths are based on the chemical principle: "the weak will draw from the strong." The hot water bathing solution draws toxins out of the body to the surface of the skin. Then, as the water cools, the toxins are pulled from the surface of the skin by the change in temperature and go into the water. The purification is brought about by the simple principle of nature that the weak (cool water) energy draws from the strong (body heated by the hot water).

It is important to remain in the bath until the water cools in order to receive the full effect of these detoxifying therapeutic baths. Adding cold water to speed up the cooling of the bath water will change the chemistry of the bath, so that is not advised.

Important: If you are pregnant, please seek the advice of your health care professional before taking any of these therapeutic baths. Consult your health care professional about the appropriateness of these baths for children.

A general caution: If you are in generally poor health, you may have to adjust the timing of these baths to make them tolerable to your system. The Parcells therapeutic baths are powerful detoxifying natural remedies; if your system is quite sensitive from the effects of chronic illnesses and drugs used to treat them, you may find it uncomfortable and unpleasant to stay in the baths for more than ten or fifteen minutes. In that case, it is best to work up to a full therapeutic bath over several bathing sessions.

THE FOUR PARCELLS THERAPEUTIC BATHING FORMULAS

Formula 1

WHEN TO DO IT   If you have been exposed to environmental radiation or X rays. Air travel, for instance, will greatly increase levels of radiation in our bodies; even simple dental X rays will leave deposits in the body that will interfere with healthy functioning.

Indications: general muscle aches, mild nausea, more fatigue than usual, headaches, slight dizziness, the discomforts associated with jet lag, or a disturbance in balance.

HOW TO DO IT   Dissolve 1 pound of sea salt or rock salt and 1 pound of baking soda in a tub of water as hot as can be tolerated. Stay in the bath until the water has cooled.

Mix ½ teaspoon of rock salt and ½ teaspoon of baking soda in a glass of warm water and sip this during the bath. Do not shower for at least four hours following the bath.

Formula 2

WHEN TO DO IT   If you have been exposed to heavy metals, such as aluminum, or to carbon monoxide or unburned carbons, pesticide sprays, or deterrents. Cooking with aluminum will bring on symptoms. Frequent commuters absorb carbon monoxide through the skin, which then gets inside the body. Eating foods that have not been cleaned of pesticides can lead to accumulations of pesticides in the cells.

Indications: a general feeling of being "out of sorts," decreased energy, upper respiratory discomfort, a shortness of breath, light-headedness, or impaired balance.

HOW TO DO IT   Add 1 cup of regular-brand Clorox® bleach (with the blue and white label) to a tub of water as hot as can be tolerated. Stay in the bath until the water has cooled. Do not shower for at least four hours following the bath.

Note: When people read a recommendation like the one above—that they should actually allow *bleach* to touch their skin—their eyebrows go up. Rest assured, the amount of bleach recommended here, in a solution of this much water, cannot hurt you. In fact, it can and will remove toxins with utmost effectiveness because it is a powerful oxygenator. You'll feel the difference in a matter of hours.

Be sensible, of course—don't use more bleach than is recommended. But do be adventurous. Try it!

Formula 3

WHEN TO DO IT   If you have been exposed to low-grade radioactive materials in the atmosphere or food irradiated by cobalt 60. In supermarkets (or in health food stores, for that matter) we usually are not told which foods are and which are not irradiated with deadly cobalt 60. Assume its residues are in a wide range of foods from fresh fruits and vegetables to grains and packaged meats.

Indications: a soreness of the gums, mouth, or throat, swollen glands, indigestion, or an inability to retain food comfortably in the stomach.

HOW TO DO IT   Dissolve 2 pounds of baking soda in a tub of water as hot as can be tolerated. Stay in the bath until the water has cooled.

Mix ½ teaspoon of baking soda in a glass of warm water and sip on this during the bath. Do not shower for at least four hours following the bath.

Formula 4

WHEN TO DO IT   This bath is a general detoxifier. It is particularly useful in raising the acid level in the body to help build immunity and ward off a feeling that you are about to be ill.

Indications: general muscle aches and pains, fatigue brought about by physical exertion, or mental or emotional stress, symptoms usually associated with the start of a cold or flu.

HOW TO DO IT   Add 2 cups of apple cider vinegar (pure, not the "flavored" variety) to a tub of water as hot as can be tolerated. Stay in the bath until the water has cooled.

Mix 1 tablespoon of apple cider vinegar into a glass of warm water and sip on this during the bath. Do not shower for at least four hours following the bath.

> *Ofttimes his [Archimedes'] servants got him against his will to the baths, to wash and anoint him: and yet being there, he would ever be drawing out of the geometrical figures, even in the very embers of the chimney. And while they were anointing of him with oils and sweet savours, with his fingers he did draw lines upon his naked body: so far was he taken from himself, and brought into an ecstasy or trance, with the delight he had in the study of geometry.*
>
> Plutarch, in *Lives,* first century A.D.

Some Points to Keep in Mind

- Therapeutic bathing is most effective before bedtime, because the body detoxifies naturally during sleep.

- Use only one bathing formula per evening.

- Do not mix ingredients from different formulas; each bath is recommended only for the specific indications described.

- The baths can be continued without harm until relief from the symptoms occurs.

- If redness, dryness, or roughness of the skin develops, it is an indication that the body is working to remove toxins. These aspects of cleansing are not uncommon. To minimize discomfort, rub a little olive or almond oil or a non-petroleum-based baby lotion on the skin after bathing.

- If you feel you have need for all the baths, alternate them on different evenings.

Caution: if these baths are in any way too rigorous or unpleasant, please use common sense and cut back application or discontinue.

THERAPEUTIC BATHING
AS NATURE'S LUXURY

The best attitude to take toward therapeutic bathing is that it is something quite special given to us by nature to help us get back to or remain in good health. Native Americans in the part of the country where Dr. Parcells grew up considered therapeutic bathing so important that they incorporated it into their religious rituals. Hot springs all over the country have been sources of physical and spiritual renewal for successive generations of Native Americans and, after them, wave after wave of newcomers.

Luxury as only nature can provide surrounds us when we bathe. We came from water, and now we go back into the water to recover life, sustenance, and the joy of health.

You can make your therapeutic bathing into your own personal ritual. Darken the room. Burn incense, if you like. Light candles. Use the time in the tub to meditate, to listen to an inspirational tape, to think (or to allow your mind to be blissfully blank). Your rituals will create a cradle of healing for yourself.

WHAT YOU CAN DO TODAY FOR BETTER HEALTH

- Become aware of toxins in almost every area of everyday life—radiation, irradiation residues, X rays, low-level radiation, pesticides, carbon monoxide—and take steps to avoid exposure to them.

- If an X ray is absolutely essential, be sure to take a therapeutic bath immediately afterward.

- Make the Parcells Method of Therapeutic Bathing part of your normal health and grooming regime.

- Consider making a ritual of therapeutic baths, creating health in the most natural way by returning to the birthing waters of our origins.

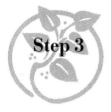

Step 3

FULL-ENERGY FUEL

If you take your foot off the brake, your car will start moving. When the body is rid of the toxins that have clogged its smooth operation, it can begin to accept nutrient-rich food and start to live fully in health.

The cornerstone of the Parcells Method of natural self-healing is simply this: if you put good, clean, usable food and water into a clean, nutrient-receptive body, you will create good health.

DR. HAZEL PARCELLS

BASIC PRINCIPLES

Dr. Parcells developed the food and water cleansings described in the following pages over two decades of research and experimentation, and many hundreds of her students can attest to their efficacy. Some of the natural treatments may sound simple—after all, just about everything she recommended for use in regaining and remaining in health is at hand in the kitchen cabinet or under the bathroom sink. So much of what she advised for good health was based on elementary information.

Although the information she worked with certainly is elementary, it is grounded on the principles of nature, which are ancient and unchanging—but which have, unfortunately, been largely forgotten.

A century ago, all food was "natural" and "organic." It was grown in soil that contained and imparted valuable nutrients to the food. The air was clean and contained all the necessary oxygen to enhance and support life. Water was plentiful and contained the natural elements required for sustenance.

A mere hundred years later, everything in our environment has changed, and we find ourselves existing in a survival mode on a planet robbed of much of its life-giving capability. Now if we are to live in health, we have to adopt new habits to meet the new problems we face.

CLEAN FOOD

The Most Effective Food Cleanser

A simple rinsing in water won't remove the poisonous residues on our food, but there is something we can use to clean foods, and chances are you have it right at hand in your kitchen cupboard or under your sink. People are usually startled when it is suggested that the best cleanser for food is household bleach.

Bleach and Old Lemons

The idea of using bleach to clean food occurred to Dr. Parcells when she was teaching nutrition and doing research at Sierra States University in California in the early 1950s. After one of her classes, a student brought her a big box full of discolored, shriveled lemons. They were "culls," or discards, fit to be thrown out, really. Dr. Parcells was delighted with them. It was the perfect opportunity for her to test a new theory she had been working on.

She filled a sink with water, put in a small amount of Clorox® bleach, and dumped the lemons in. It wasn't long before the fragrance of lemons filled the whole area. Half an hour later, when she went back to check the sink, the lemons had taken on a fresh appearance. The discoloration and shrinkage were gone. These were new, bright yellow lemons, as fresh looking as if they had been picked from the tree that very day.

Dr. Parcells wondered what she would do with all these lemons after they had been restored to their original quality. That is when they ceased being just lemons and became a key ingredient for scientific investigation.

She separated them into portions and stored them in a freezer where, for the next three years, they were tested for freshness and nutritional value in every class. And at the last class they were as full of life-sustaining energy as at the first. They retained their freshness, moisture, and tart flavor and proved to be an adequate rival to the naturally fresh fruit brought in for comparison.

What had happened was this: the sodium hypochlorite in the Clorox® bleach, a natural oxygenator, apparently set up an action with the natural chemicals in the lemons, making them "fresh" again. Subsequent tests showed the Clorox® bleach also cleaned the lemons, eliminating any type of fungus, bacteria, or other foreign material on them that might have contributed to a disorder or to earlier than usual deterioration.

Most bleaches on the market use the same or a similar chemical formula, but, after many tests, Dr. Parcells found that the original Clorox® bleach was the best to use for cleansing purposes. She attributed the success of Clorox® bleach for food cleansing to the maker's superior filtration systems and high quality of manufacture.

That was the beginning of Dr. Parcells's research into restoring vitality to foods. Over the next few years she continued her experiments, refined her methods, and shared them with people who were concerned about the devitalizing effects of chemicals on the food supply.

Household Bleach Is Not Chlorine

Household bleach is not chlorine, even though some call it "chlorine bleach." It's no more chlorine than is common table salt (sodium chloride). And when used in the home and disposed of down the household drain, it's no more harmful to the environment than salt. It is true that chlorine is used in the manufacturing of household bleach, but the end product contains no free chlorine. Bleach is produced by combining chlorine and caustic soda (sodium hydroxide). In the process, the two ingredients completely convert into a new product—sodium hypochlorite, the active ingredient in household bleach. Inside a Clorox® bleach bottle is a 5.25 percent solution of sodium hypochlorite and water.

The Bleach Cycle: Salt Water to Salt Water

1. Chlorine manufacturers produce chlorine and sodium hydroxide by running an electric current through salt water.

2. The Clorox Company purchases chlorine and makes household bleach by bubbling it into a solution of water and sodium hydroxide. During this process, all of the chlorine is converted to a sodium hypochlorite solution.

3. Household bleach is produced—a 5.25 percent solution of hypochlorite and water.

4. During use as a cleaner and disinfectant, and during disposal, about 95 to 98 percent of the bleach quickly breaks down into salt.

5. The remaining 2 to 5 percent of the bleach breaks down to form by-products that are effectively treated at municipal wastewater treatment plants or septic systems through biodegradation.

6. By the end of the cycle, the sodium hypochlorite has once again become salt.

(Source: Information from the Clorox Company. For more information write The Clorox Company, Oakland, CA 94612, or phone 1–800–292–2808. Also see the company's web page: www.clorox.com.)

Disclaimer

During her research into the oxidizing effects of Clorox® bleach on foods, Dr. Parcells never approached the Clorox Company for any reason; she never asked for either consent or advice. The Clorox Company is in no way responsible for the information on the use of the product in these cleansing soaks.

The Parcells Oxygen Soak

The Parcells Oxygen Soak method of cleaning food is good for all food items that can be immersed in water, including most fruits and vegetables, many grains, legumes, meats, poultry, and fish.

Eggs are at the top of the list of allergy-causing foods. This may be due to the pesticide sprays used around chicken cages and nests. The eggshell is porous and can absorb these poisons very quickly.

Salmonella bacteria may also be present in eggs, as they are often found in the chickens themselves.

By putting eggs into the Clorox® bleach soak, you will find they have a better flavor and will have lost their tendency to cause allergies.

Meat is one of the heaviest carriers of toxic materials. It contains residues of the growth hormones and antibiotic shots injected directly into animals, plus the poisons in the food they consume. By placing meats in the cleansing soak, the poisonous substances will be eliminated, the flavor of the meat will be improved, and the tissue will be tenderized. This applies to all flesh foods, including fish, which usually contains a considerable amount of mercury and many other toxic materials.

If the meat is frozen, it will not lose any of its juices when placed in the Clorox® bleach soak. Any frozen meat, turkey, fish, or chicken can remain in the soak until thawed. All meats except the ground varieties can be treated in the cleansing soak—and even these may be treated if they are not too loose to begin with.

Dr. Parcells's procedures were developed and tested during several years of research. She used the Clorox® bleach food cleansing method for forty years and never had a complaint from anyone who adopted it—nor was there an unsatisfactory reaction of any kind. In fact, everyone who has used this method of cleansing agrees that food tastes better, keeps longer, remains fresher, and, most important, sustains better health.

> *A very educated man came to see me. He had heard about the miracles my cleansing methods performed turning lifeless, contaminated substances into excellent quality food. I told him how he could clean his food by putting it into a solution of water with a few drops of Clorox® bleach.*

> *"But bleach is a poison!"* he exclaimed.
> *"A spoonful of whisky won't kill you,"* I said, *"but a quart might."* I never heard from him again. There is no use in trying to educate the overeducated; they've already made up their minds about how things work.
>
> Dr. Hazel Parcells

Step-by-Step Method for Cleaning Foods

Formula: Make the Parcells Oxygen Soak by adding 1 teaspoon of Clorox® bleach to 1 gallon of water.

Separate food to be cleaned into the following groups:

Vegetables:
> *Leafy vegetables*
> *Root and heavy-fiber vegetables*

Fruits:
> *Thin-skinned fruits, such as berries*
> *Medium-skinned fruits, such as peaches, apricots, plums*
> *Thick-skinned fruits, such as apples*
> *Citrus fruits and bananas*

Eggs

Meat/poultry

Soak: Into the solution place the fruits, vegetables, or other foods to be treated. Refer to the following timing chart, because timing is very important. Make a fresh soak for each group.

Leafy vegetables	*5–10 min.*
Root and heavy-fiber vegetables	*10–15 min.*

Thin-skinned berries	*5 min.*
Medium-skinned fruits	*10 min.*
Thick-skinned fruits	*10–15 min.*
Citrus fruits and bananas	*15 min.*
Eggs	*20–30 min.*
Meats/poultry per pound (thawed)	*10 min.*
Meats/poultry per pound (frozen)	*15–20 min.*

Some people are concerned that soaking vegetables, for instance, will cause them to lose their mineral content. This cannot happen in 15 to 30 minutes. The mineral activity is only increased, as you will discover.

Do *not* use more Clorox® bleach than instructed, and do not leave food in the soak longer than the suggested time. If left too long in the solution, green leafy vegetables will turn brown from oxidation. No harm is done, but the eye appeal is spoiled.

Rinse: After the soak, remove the food and place it in a fresh water rinse for 5 to 10 minutes. This is an important step, because the fresh water introduces a flood of new oxygen into the food.

Store: Now the food is ready to be prepared for storage. Let the food drain very well before placing it in the refrigerator.

The Benefits of Cleaning Food Using the Parcells Oxygen Soak

The benefits of the oxygen food treatment are many. Fruits and vegetables will keep longer. The wilted ones will return to a fresh crispness. Drained, faded hues will give way to vivid, vibrant colors; tastelessness will be replaced with flavor and tang. For very little effort, you will have fresh, crunchy vegetables and juicy, sweet, zesty fruits that will keep twice as long.

With the cleansing soak, the flavors of both fruits and vegetables will be enhanced greatly—they will taste as fresh as if they had just been picked from the garden or the orchard. Most important, once the food is cleansed, all the dangerous additives in it will have been removed.

Remember to use only original Clorox® bleach for the cleansing soaks.

The Parcells Oxygen Soak has been used around the world with great success—particularly in many developing countries. It has been adopted by health departments of governments. People who have been in the Peace Corps or diplomatic service will recognize it as the essential means of sanitizing food in out-of-the-way places.

The Parcells Method formula is also registered with the Smithsonian Institution as an exhibit under "Simplified Kitchen Chemistry."

CLEAN WATER

So much for food—but what about water?

If you thought you could never have really fresh, clean drinking water—in spite of all the filtered, treated, and bottled water out there—you haven't heard about the Parcells method of cleaning plain, ordinary tap water.

There *is* a way to drink healthy water all the time. It's safe, easy, inexpensive, and completely effective.

Tap water that is put under a *full-spectrum light* will be cleaned of all harmful materials—and will taste wonderful.

The Water Problem

Water is the principal constituent of our bodies, comprising about 75 percent of what we are. It is necessary for all metabolic functions within cells, since it is the medium in which chemical re-actions operate. Water is, in short, the indispensable fluid of our existence.

Over the years, Dr. Parcells traced the seemingly incurable conditions of many of her clients to the water they were drinking. Even after stoking their bodies with the missing ingredients their systems needed to utilize the food inside to optimum effect, she would still encounter the presence of virulent poisons.

She began looking into the water supply in the home. Her work was often with families, and when the same condition showed up in an entire family, it had to be caused by something of which they all partook. The same principle can be applied to whole communities, by the way; it is not uncommon for outbreaks of disease to be traced to a water supply contaminated with parasites and bacteria.

Her research revealed many hidden problems and resolved many previously unanswered questions. She found that those of her clients who were using distilled water and water treated with water softeners for drinking and cooking showed definite muscle weakness, particularly of the heart, one of the first places poor mineral balance manifests itself. Also, in the same people, general muscle tone throughout the body was very poor. And the blood chemistry of the users of distilled and softened water showed significant deficiencies in calcium and other important supportive minerals.

It was apparent that it would be a real problem to get the needed nutrients that should be supplied in water and at the same time dispel the accumulation of poisons that are ever present in ordinary drinking water.

Tap Water

Tap water, unless it is piped in from a well in the backyard, is universally suspect as a healthy drink, and rightly so. Municipal water supplies are treated in various ways in many parts of the country, which is why "city water" tastes somewhat different from place to place. But all city water is treated to kill bacteria. The agents of killing—"purifying" is the euphemism used—are manufactured chemicals designed expressly to be fatal to living microorganisms. Such a public health precaution would be fine, except that many bacteria are not only helpful, but also necessary for the human body to function at top form. Without them we are prey to all kinds of subtle malfunctions, particularly in digestion. Poor digestion will eventually lead to a general breakdown of health.

Vital minerals are also screened out in most municipal water supplies. The few waterborne living minerals left undissolved by chemicals are caught by filters before drinking water is allowed to flow to homes. The result, by any means of measurement, is lifeless water.

A curious note: water without *any* bacterial content can nevertheless carry common communicable diseases, perhaps because no bacteria are present to combat them. Some years ago, when Dr. Parcells lived in Albuquerque, she regularly tested the drinking water whenever epidemics of influenza, measles, or chicken pox broke out in the schools. As she suspected, she found those germs thriving in tap water.

In her classes, Dr. Parcells always tested drinking water brought to her by students. Water out of home faucets invariably had a reading of 15 on her life-energy scale;* a reading of 120 is needed to support normal body function.

---

*Dr. Parcells used an energy scale that went from 0 to 360 degrees. She obtained readings by using a specially made pendulum. Step Seven will go into this in much more detail.

> *Two major environmental groups [have] released studies assert-ing that more than one-fifth of the U.S. population drink tap water contaminated by lead, fecal bacteria, toxic waste, and other pollutants.*
>
> *The groups—the Natural Resources Defense Council and the Environmental Working Group—based their studies on 1993–94 statistics released by the Environmental Protection Agency and information from local water utilities. Both groups concluded that 53 million people in the U.S. in 1993 and 1994 were drinking water that did not meet quality standards set by the Clean Water Act. That marked a 7.6-million-person increase over the figure for 1991–92.*
>
> *According to the groups, consumption of contaminated water annually caused between 1,000 and 1,200 deaths and more than seven million cases of mild to moderate illness.*
>
> *The reports indicated that individuals with compromised immune systems, such as people with AIDS or those undergoing cancer chemotherapy treatment, were particularly vulnerable to waterborne illnesses.*
>
> *The EWG study reported that disease-causing fecal coliform bacteria, which was commonly found in sewage, was present in 1,172 water systems that supplied drinking water to 11.6 million people across the U.S.*
>
> *Facts on File, June 8, 1995*

- In 1995 the Environmental Protection Agency (EPA) and the Centers for Disease Control and Prevention (CDC) issued a report warning that drinking tap water could be life-threatening to the five million Americans with weakened immune systems.

- The EPA estimates that about 30 million Americans a year are drinking from public water systems that violate one or more health standards.

- Researchers at the Medical College of Wisconsin in Milwaukee found that people who regularly drink tap water containing high levels of chlorine by-products have a greater risk of developing bladder and rectal cancers than people who drink unchlorinated water.

- Because cryptosporidium was only recently recognized as a [health] threat and tests are unreliable, there are no laws requiring utilities to check specifically for the parasite.

Adapted from Deborah Kotz, "How Safe Is Your Water?" *Good Housekeeping*, November 1995

Tap Water Contaminants Glossary

Cysts: the form in which intestinal parasites, such as cryptosporidium and giardia, exist outside the body.

Atrazine, chlordane, lindane, toxaphene: pesticides.

Particulates: dirt and sediment.

Turbidity: a state of cloudiness that often signals microbiological contamination.

VOCs (volatile organic compounds): a class of chemicals that includes chlorine by-products.

Chlorine has proven to be a helpful disinfectant for drinking water, having been used to neutralize bacteria and other waterborne pathogens since 1908 in the United States. In the 1970s,

> *however, it was discovered that chemicals left in the water from contact with soil and decaying vegetation were reacting with chlorine to create "disinfection by-products," such as chloroform. Disinfection by-products may cause more than 10,000 rectal and bladder cancers each year in the United States and may also be linked to pancreatic cancer and birth defects. To keep these by-products from forming, water companies must remove organic materials prior to chlorination, by filtration or other means, or switch to disinfectants that cause fewer problems.*
>
> Adapted from Scott Alan Lewis, "Trouble on Tap," in *Sierra*, July-August 1995

Bottled, Filtered, and Distilled Water

But what about bottled water? The dedicated person lugging several large containers into the health food store to fill up on filtered, reverse-osmosis, distilled, or spring water surely is getting all the health benefits of good, pure water, right? The diner in a fancy restaurant ordering a bottle of expensive "designer" spring water is choosing a healthy alternative to tap water, true?

False. Bottled water is still the water of our planet, and our planet's environment is despoiled. Chemical fertilizers, radiation, pesticides, the wastes of a century of wars, the emissions from the burning of fossil fuels—all of these are in the atmosphere. And if they are in our air, they are also in our water. With very few exceptions (such as exceptionally pure water from aquifers that filter by a natural process in the earth), all our water is contaminated—even if it ends up in a bottle with an elegant label.

Distilled water has no life-energy at all. To test this in the kitchen, pour distilled water into a teapot that has built up a residue of crusty white minerals and chemicals around the inside and leave it overnight. In the morning the water (which is "empty" of life and therefore draws life to itself) will have soaked up the residue.

Distilled water does have uses in health enhancement: Dr. Parcells used it in some of her fasting programs to sponge up toxins in the body. But used as drinking water, it is entirely useless, even health-compromising.

Filtered water presents problems of its own. First, while impurities are filtered out of the water, valuable minerals are also taken out at the same time. Second, the filter collects impurities, so the more the filter is used, the worse the water is for having gone through a filthy filter.

The Solution

Dr. Parcells experimented with many different approaches to solve the drinking water problem. Finally she found a solution. All life on our planet depends for nourishment on light from the sun, a critical balance of visible color and invisible ultraviolet wavelengths. Virtually every living thing has developed with the aid of nature's full spectrum of light. The essence of life in energy is . . . color.

Full-spectrum lights have the same effect as the light from the sun, which is vital to life and health. They contain, as the name implies, the energy from the entire spectrum of light given off by the sun—and natural sunlight is, of course, one of nature's oldest cures.

When Dr. Parcells first experimented with full-spectrum lighting on tap water, she was quite surprised. The rays of light cleaned the water totally of germs and chemical additives and revived the content of its original energy. In a short time, "dead" water came fully to life.

In her school in Los Angeles, and later in Albuquerque, she installed a full-spectrum light in the kitchen under the cupboard over the counter. Four one-gallon glass jars of tap water were under the light at all times. As she and her students would finish one gallon of full-spectrum water, they would refill the jar and place it at the back of the line. The water was clean, flavorful, and life-giving. It was their water for drinking, cooking, and watering pets and plants.

> *While doing some time-lapse photography for Walt Disney, [John] Ott observed that pumpkin seed sprouts would not fully mature under fluorescent lights, but that they flourished if ultraviolet light was added to the light source. Following years of study of the effects of different light sources on plants, he turned his attention to the question of their effects on animals.*
>
> *Based on the results of these and other studies, Ott . . . recommended to Duro-Test Corporation that it modify one of its fluorescent tubes to more closely replicate the full spectrum of natural sunlight. He suggested that they do this by adding a phosphor that would produce the three types of ultraviolet radiation in the same proportions as they are present in sunlight. Through the investigations, suggestions, and inspiration of Ott, Duro-Test succeeded in developing the first full-spectrum fluorescent tube, the Vita-Lite.*
>
> Jacob Liberman, in *Light: Medicine of the Future,* 1991

How to Clean Your Drinking Water

You too can clean the water in your own home. Forget filtered water and distilled water, which can impart no life-energy because they have no energy to begin with.

To clean your tap water, fill a gallon glass container with water from the tap and place it directly under a full-spectrum light. The light should be no more than a foot away from the water. It will take approximately thirty minutes to clean the water. The light can be attached under a kitchen cabinet to shine down on a countertop, as was done in the original experiments of Dr. Parcells.

> *Once, a little girl dying of anemia was brought to me. After researching the matter, I found that the water the family was drinking was highly infused with arsenic. They lived close to a large farm. The arsenic had come from seepage from the irrigation where pesticides and herbicides had been applied. The arsenic had not affected other members of the family—at least not yet. But the little girl's immune system was quite depressed, and the arsenic was eroding her health away.*
>
> *I recommended that the family move, but they couldn't do it for economic reasons. So I suggested they clean their water with a full-spectrum light. That was something they could do. In a month's time, the child's anemia completely disappeared.*
>
> Dr. Hazel Parcells

Full-Spectrum Lighting

Full-spectrum light is the synthetic version of the sun's own light. In concentrated form, as light containing the full spectrum of color from the sun, it is a powerful cleansing agent.

Full-spectrum light bulbs are long tubes that look like fluorescent bulbs. They give off a soft glow.

An enlightened hardware store or a health food store in your neighborhood probably carries full-spectrum lights. If not, ask the store to order them for you.

Dr. Parcells experimented with several brands of full-spectrum lights and found one to be particularly effective. Parcells Center will direct you to it.

Parcells Center
P.O. Box 2129
Santa Fe, NM 87504–2129
1–800–811–6784

The Benefits of Cleaning Contaminated Water

It's gratifying to see the recovery of entire families from a chronic health disturbance once their water supply is cleaned up. Dr. Parcells helped one family in California in which every member had one type of infection or another all the time, with some members continually in the hospital. The mother was having a great deal of skin trouble, with burning and swelling of the hands and face; a rash had spread over her entire body like a severe reaction to a poison.

After Dr. Parcells investigated the family's water supply—the last resort, she recorded in her notes—she found the culprit. Their water came from a shallow well into which had seeped an accumulation of liquids carrying commercial fertilizers used in the gardens and orchards that surrounded the house.

When the well water was analyzed, all of the gram-negative bacteria were found, as well as many of the bacteria prevailing in common physical disorders. Everything but the Black Plague was there. When the water supply was cleaned up under full-spectrum lights, the family's health problems ended.

Another outstanding case involved a client who suffered miserably from severe muscle pains that could not be alleviated. Dr. Parcells found that the woman's entire muscle structure was heavily impregnated with highly toxic mercury. She had no record of being exposed to mercury, so the next step was to check the water supply. Mercury was found in her drinking water in exactly the same proportion as that in her muscle structure. After cleaning the water supply with full-spectrum lighting, the problem vanished and the woman regained her energy and freedom from pain.

Could it be so simple? You can try it for yourself and see that it really works.

WHAT YOU CAN DO TODAY
FOR BETTER HEALTH

• Clean all food coming into the home that can be immersed in water in the Parcells Oxygen Soak: 1 teaspoon of regular-brand Clorox® bleach to 1 gallon of water. Soak according to the time chart provided in this section and rinse in clear water afterward. The oxygen soak will remove all dangerous chemicals, the effects of radiation, and all other toxic substances from food and will reoxygenate it, giving you the benefits of food that is both clean and nutritionally useful.

• Clean all water for cooking and drinking under a full-spectrum light. Place a gallon jug of tap water under a full-spectrum light for thirty minutes. The full-spectrum light treatment will clean water of dangerous bacteria, chemicals, and pollutants and enliven it with energy.

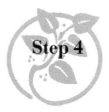

Step 4

OPTIMUM ASSIMILATION

Even the highest quality food can't be used properly unless it is well digested and becomes an energy-efficient part of ourselves.

Some foods combine well with others for best digestion; some foods, mixed with others at the same meal, will cause indigestion and, worse, as time goes on and toxins are accumulated in the body, severe and irreversible health problems.

When you know something about the chemistry of foods, you have in your own hands the power over your health.

DR. HAZEL PARCELLS

THE FOOD WE EAT

Food Combining for Best Digestion

How we eat our food is as important to good health as *what* we eat. We are speaking here about combining food for proper digestion—and remember that the digestion of food and the absorption of its life force form the most direct route to gaining and remaining in health.

Much has been written on the subject of food combining. Dr. Parcells found the great bulk of it to be of little worth. So much of the literature on food and nutrition is confusing, contradictory, and downright incorrect. Some authors of diet books tell us that we can't hang onto life unless we eat only fruit in the morning. Others say we'll faint dead away by noon if we don't eat good hearty proteins in the morning.

Common sense often takes the back seat when it comes to matters of nutrition. This is peculiar, since one might think the easiest and most natural thing in the world for us to do, as living human animals, is to eat food. But we have built walls of ignorance and impracticality around the subject that are very hard to scale.

Dr. Parcells studied the chemistry of foods for more than sixty years and applied her knowledge with excellent results. In all that time she saw literally scores of different eating plans and heard arguments on many different sides of the major nutritional questions. Sorting through the volumes of material was often an exasperating experience for her—but it also was instructive.

As you might imagine by now, she had very little patience with unrealistic approaches to living—and food is the most basic element of living we know of. What Dr. Parcells discovered about food combining for good health can be boiled down to three simple rules—which are nature's own rules. If you adopt them as your eating habits, you'll be able to tell the difference in the way you feel and look and the way you use the energy you bring to life.

Proteins	Starches
Beef	Breads
Lamb	Cornmeal
Veal	Light-colored beans
Pork	Flour and all flour products
Poultry	Hominy
Fish	Pasta
Eggs	Oatmeal
Milk	Potatoes
Cheese	Rice
Cottage cheese	Yellow split peas
Nuts	Most grains
Dark-colored beans	
Some grains	

Food-Combining Recommendations

RECOMMENDATION ONE   *Eat only one protein at a meal.*

Avoid combining two proteins at the same meal, for example, steak with lobster, or chicken with ham, or beef with bacon.

This recommendation extends not only to meat and poultry proteins, but also other proteins such as legumes and dairy products. Thus, beans are incompatible with pork, and a glass of milk with a hamburger is a poor food combination. Mixing proteins will lead to digestive problems and have a negative impact on total health.

The only exception to the one-protein recommendation is eggs, which combine well with anything.

High-protein grains, such as "hard" or "winter" wheat, do not combine well with other proteins. Dark beans contain more protein than starch and therefore do not mix well with other proteins.

Eating two proteins at the same meal will result in poor digestion because each protein requires a different chemical process for breakdown and absorption. Foods that are not completely digested linger in the body and putrefy, creating toxins. An accumulation of toxins in the body will eventually lead to health problems.

RECOMMENDATION TWO   *Eat meat, poultry, and fish separate from dairy products.*

At the same meal, avoid combining meat, poultry, and fish with dairy products. Cheese and meats together (cheeseburgers, for example) are practically indigestible—as are other similar combinations: fish with a cheese sauce, turkey with cottage cheese, beef with an ice-cream dessert.

Dairy products high in fat should be considered *fats*, not dairy; a butter sauce on fish, for instance, is a proper combination. The same holds true for a sauce made with cream; it may enhance the flavor of well-prepared meat and poultry, and, since it is more fat than dairy, the combination will not interfere with good digestion.

Dairy products are difficult for the human system to digest under any circumstances. However, dairy combined with green leafy vegetables (cheese on salads, for instance) is an appropriate mixture. Other, nonstarchy vegetables go well with dairy products (broccoli with a cheese sauce, for instance), but care should be taken not to combine vegetables that are mostly starch with dairy products. A baked potato with a sour-cream topping, for example, will not digest well; a baked potato with butter is a much better digestive mix.

Milk on cereal is not a good nutritional idea, since the digestive juices necessary to break down the milk for assimilation are not the same needed to alter starches for digestion. Cream on cooked cereal creates a good mix for digestion. Yogurt with fruit is a reasonably good combination.

RECOMMENDATION THREE   *Eat meat, poultry, fish, and dairy products separate from most starches.*

At the same meal, avoid mixing meat, poultry, or fish with gluten-based starches such as wheat, rye, oats, barley—that is, all bread, pastries, cereals, and pastas.

Such non-gluten-based vegetable starches as potatoes, corn, rice, peas, and millet will combine well with animal proteins *provided a green leafy vegetable is included in the meal.*

A meat-and-bread sandwich will not digest well; meat *or* cheese on a corn tortilla, which is made from a non-gluten-based vegetable starch, is a much better combination—when accompanied by a green leafy vegetable.

Milk is an animal protein and is digested as a protein. Cream, however, is essentially an animal fat and is digested as a fat. So, milk on hot cereal will present a digestive problem, but cream on hot cereal will digest well.

A word about wheat. Athough wheat is a staple of the American diet, it should be treated with respect. The several varieties of wheat are hearty fare in themselves and as such will not combine well with many other foods. Many people are actually allergic to wheat without knowing it—and the origin of their trouble, ironically, may be in wheat's own nourishing quality, which prevents it from mixing well with other foods, especially proteins.

Wheat does appear to combine well with vegetables. Vegetable soup with wheat bread or crackers will digest well; beef soup and chicken soup do not combine well with wheat (especially "hard" or "winter" wheat) bread.

The Three Food-Combining Recommendations

1. Eat only one protein at a meal. The exception: eggs, which combine well with everything.

2. Eat meat, poultry, and fish separate from dairy products.

3. Eat meat, poultry, fish, and dairy products separate from most starches.

Eat Simple

One further note. It is not a rule, but a general approach to eating for optimum digestion: try to limit the *kinds* of foods eaten at one meal to as few as possible. Instead of going for the highest diversity, strive for simplicity. "Surf-and-turf" dishes are indigestible, but a simple meal of fish with a salad and steamed vegetables is life-giving. Several-course meals may look good, but, unless combined scrupulously, they are more about quantity than quality and have nothing to do with real nourishment.

A bowl of cooked oatmeal and a piece of fruit is a meal. A piece of chicken and a spinach salad is a meal. Going in the direction of ever more variety in a single meal can be disastrous for digestion. Staying simple within the confines of a meal will yield huge benefits in digestion and in total health.

Dr. Parcells lived by the three general recommendations for food combining for more than sixty years. As you can see, they are quite elementary and, if you know a little about food chemistry, quite logical. Keeping these rules kept Dr. Parcells and all those who came to her for help in good health.

Mary had a little lamb,
A lobster and some prunes,
A glass of milk, a piece of pie,
And then some macaroons.
It made the naughty waiters grin
To see her order so;
And when they carried Mary out
Her face was white as snow.

This little lamb that Mary had,
It followed where she went,
Along with nuts and cheese; of, sad
To say, on mischief bent.
It made poor Mary groan and jump
And twitch and squirm and shout.
They had to use the stomach pump
To bail poor Mary out.

"What makes lamb do Mary so?"
The eager nurses cry.
'Cause Mary mixed her lamb, you know,
With cider and mince pie,
And other things too numerous
To mention in this poem.
Take my advice: don't mix your foods
As through this world you roam.

Though Mary loved her lamb, you bet,
A solemn oath she swore:

*To ne'er mix lamb with her spaghet
And lobster anymore.
And always as the years passed by,
When she was asked to state
What else she'll have, she would reply:
"I'll take my lambkin straight."*

Anonymous, quoted in George Albert Wilson,
A New Slant to Diet, 1950

Planning Meals

The following procedure will help you obtain the best possible nutritional advantage from your food.

During a day, it is best to eat one predominantly starch (complex carbohydrate) meal, one fruit or green vegetable meal, and one protein-and-vegetable meal.

Usually the starch meal, which is a "heat" meal, provides a good breakfast: cooked whole-grain cereals, breads, hotcakes, and the like. These are especially good for children, who are quite active, and people who do heavy physical work.

A fresh-fruit or green-vegetable salad makes an excellent lunch. One protein can be added to a salad, but be sure not to mix two or more proteins. A fruit salad with cheese or cottage cheese *or* nuts is a fine combination; a fresh garden salad with cold fish *or* meat *or* poultry and a dressing of olive oil and apple cider vinegar or lemon juice is a wonderful midday meal.

For dinner, cooked vegetables, a raw vegetable salad, and a protein dish make a filling and nutritious meal. For the most nourishing and efficient vitamin and mineral diversification, include in the meal two vegetables that grow *above* the ground and one that grows *below:* spinach, cauliflower, and carrots, for instance, or broccoli, endive, and potatoes.

Sample Menus

Sample menu for a person doing light work or trying to lose weight:

Breakfast: Fresh fruit juice (30 min. before other food)
                     [mineral salts]
                 1 egg, soft-boiled or poached [protein]
                 1 bran muffin [carbohydrate]
                 1 pat butter, 2 tsp. cream [hydrocarbons]
                 Coffee, tea, or other hot beverage

Lunch: 2–3 oz. cheese [protein]
                 Salad of fresh greens [mineral salts]
                 Cornbread [carbohydrate]
                 1 tbsp. olive oil and lemon juice dressing
                     [hydrocarbons]

Dinner: 4–6 oz. chicken breast (baked or poached)
                     [protein]
                 Coleslaw, olive oil and vinegar dressing
                     [mineral salts]
                 Brussels sprouts, steamed [mineral salts]
                 Carrots, steamed [mineral salts]
                 1–2 tbsp. olive oil and lemon juice dressing
                     [hydrocarbons]

Sample menu for a person doing heavy work, for children, or for a person maintaining weight:

Breakfast: Fresh fruit juice (30 min. before other food)
      [mineral salts]
      2 eggs, soft-boiled or poached [protein]
      ⅔ c. steel-cut oats [carbohydrate]
      4 prunes [carbohydrate]
      2 slices whole-wheat toast [carbohydrate]
      ¼ c. light cream [hydrocarbons]
      1 pat butter [hydrocarbons]

Lunch: 1 c. black beans or black bean soup [protein]
      Raw celery, carrots, jicama [mineral salts]
      1 c. brown rice [carbohydrate]
      Olive oil and lemon juice dressing for vegetables
      [hydrocarbons]
      Corn tortillas [carbohydrate]

Dinner: 4–6 oz. lean beef or veal [protein]
      Salad of fresh greens [mineral salts]
      1 c. beets, steamed [mineral salts]
      1 c. asparagus, steamed [mineral salts]
      1 tbsp. olive oil and lemon juice dressing
      [hydrocarbons]
      1 baked apple with cinnamon [carbohydrate]

Every Body Is Different

We are all human beings, made from the same mineral substances of the earth and therefore subject to nature's general rules, but each one of us differs from everyone else in exact body chemistry. When following the guidance suggested above, please remember to take into consideration body type, weight, height, and especially factors such as the kind of energy expenditures you make (whether they are heavy or light, physical or mental, and so on). Try various approaches for yourself in terms of quantity. Food is fuel for the body; if you don't need much fuel, don't take it in. Unspent fuel is either stored as fat or remains in the intestine, where it will spoil and become a health problem.

See how easy or how difficult it is for you to digest certain foods. Fruit, for example. There are many recommendations about fruit. One school of thought considers "acid fruits," such as oranges and grapefruits, incompatible with "sweet fruits," like bananas and papayas. Another forbids mixing fruits of any kind with other food types. Still another recommends eating only fruit until noon to wash out the digestive system.

Dr. Parcells took a more sensible approach based on her studies of food chemistry. She believed that eating fruit in combination with other food items is fine—unless the mixture upsets your stomach, causes gas, brings on indigestion, saps your energy, or makes you mentally "fuzzy." We can learn a great deal by listening to how our bodies respond to particular food types. Dr. Parcells often cooked meats with tenderizing fruit and fruit juices and had marvelous results. For others, cooking and eating meat with fruit may present a digestive problem. The key is to experiment—and to listen to what your body can handle.

Food That's Alive

Finally, let the highest and most important rule in eating for health be to begin with food that contains the life force. Starting with something packaged, processed, canned, precooked, sealed up, waxed, something that has been managed and manipulated until there's nothing left but the vague appearance of food, is asking for trouble. It is like beginning a journey with poor-quality fuel in the tank: we won't get very far down the road in that condition.

Fresh, living foods—"in season," if possible—properly cleaned and prepared, then properly combined into meals and eaten with awareness and gratitude, will provide us with excellent digestion and absorption—and good health.

THE VESSELS OF LIFE

Our forebears in ancient times took a great deal of care in the preparation of food. The utensils they left behind—beautifully crafted and colorful as well as useful—are testimony to the worth they placed on food and on the process of transforming it into nourishment for the body.

The selection of pots and pans and the other equipment we use to prepare food is every bit as significant as the choice of food we buy at the market. What we do with food in the kitchen and how we do it represent, in a nutritional sense, a life or death situation.

When you prepare food, you are a chemist, and the kitchen is your laboratory. More actual chemistry takes place in the kitchen than in any laboratory in the world. It's the heart of the home, the center of nourishment and life. The kitchen is a place where the art and science of accurate food combining come together with cooking techniques that enhance food digestion and absorption.

Food and food preparation are such a vital part of our lives and the lives of our families and loved ones that we do well to make an effort to learn some basic principles of kitchen science. Our lives quite literally depend on this knowledge.

Aluminum

The devastating consequences of using aluminum cookware cannot be overstated. Half of all cookware sold on the market is made of aluminum, which means that most households have something or other in the kitchen that is made of aluminum. Foods high in acid, such as tomato sauce, rhubarb, and sauerkraut, will oxidize aluminum, which is leached into the food cooked in those utensils and then consumed with the meal.

Water containing fluoride increases aluminum leaching. Aluminum teapots, frying pans, and kettles leave a residue in foods that, once ingested, will cause a slow poisoning of the brain, which, in extreme cases, may manifest itself as a gradual mental deterioration. Get rid of the aluminum in your kitchen as soon as possible. This includes the aluminum foil that so many people use as a disposable broiling pan or to wrap leftovers.

A few weeks after receiving a set of aluminum cookware, a patient and his wife began complaining of "feeling sick." After switching back to cooking with their stainless steel set, their complaints disappeared.

Journal of the American Medical Association, July 20, 1994

For years, researchers have puzzled over the surprisingly high levels of aluminum that turn up in the shriveled brains of Alzheimer's disease victims. While some scientists believe that the aluminum deposits are only a side effect of Alzheimer's, a growing number of investigators say that aluminum may play a central role in causing the disease.

Mark Nichols, in *Maclean's*, April 10, 1996

(It may be of interest to note that the first aluminum saucepan was invented in 1889, the year Dr. Parcells was born. However, she took no responsibility for this unhappy event.)

Graniteware

Graniteware, an old kitchen staple, is cheap, but that is about all one can say for it. If it is dropped and cracked or even a small piece of it is broken, it becomes an immediate health hazard. Since these chips and cracks may happen often, replacement eventually becomes costly. Like other thin, lightweight cookware, graniteware requires more water and higher temperatures for cooking—neither of which is recommended for the scientific preparation of food.

Glassware

Since glass does not conduct heat evenly, food is cooked above a critical temperature and thus loses many nutrients. Like graniteware, glassware has a high replacement cost, especially when used for top-of-the-stove cooking. Sometimes it will break in the oven. Like graniteware, it requires high cooking temperatures and a lot of water—two nutritional minuses. However, it is a good utensil for oven baking.

Iron Cookware

Among the oldest and most rugged in the field, iron cookware can serve in many capacities, from the broiler on the kitchen range to the campfire skillet.

The cast-iron skillet and the Dutch oven are enduring pieces of kitchen equipment. Iron conducts heat evenly and holds it well, so that the electromagnetic energies in foods are protected. Iron cookware also allows for very slow cooking, which is a tremendous plus for nutrition.

Copper Cookware

Utensils with copper bottoms are problematic: the heat stops where the copper ends; consequently the food will be hot on the bottom, but cold and uncooked on top. Copper tarnishes easily and is difficult to keep clean and in good condition. Also, copper can be toxic at much lower heat levels than aluminum.

Earthen Pots

Earthen pots, such as bean pots and casseroles, are a real joy to use. They are, of course, the most ancient of cooking utensils; using them reinforces a strong connection to the prehistoric past of our species.

When well heated, earthen pots retain an even heat and continue cooking at a very low temperature, particularly when placed in a preheated 350-degree oven that is then immediately reduced to 200 degrees. At this stage, food is cooking at 180 degrees within the pot, below a critical temperature that does not destroy the electromagnetic energy in the food.

A good bean pot is like a good friend. One has to treat it with care and respect, because replacing it can be costly. Make sure, though, that the earthenware does not contain lead, arsenic, or cadmium. If you are in doubt about its possible additives, it pays to phone the manufacturer.

Enamelware

Use caution with enamelware, as some foreign manufacturers have decorated the interior of the cookware, including the lids, with brightly colored cadmium enamels. These utensils have been banned from the United States. Many crockpots are made of enamelware. Checking the manufacturer's instructions before using is important.

"Nonstick" Cookware

Nonstick pots and pans—"miracles of the modern age"—have been shown to emit fumes fatally toxic to caged pet birds when the utensils are overheated. They can't be too much better for humans. Once the miracle coating is scratched or cracked, toxic chemicals leach into the food being cooked. Most of this coating is put over aluminum-based cookware in any case, and that is a double problem as far as nutrition goes.

Although the FDA has said about flaked pieces from nonstick surfaces, "these particles will pass unchanged through your body and pose no health hazard," there doesn't seem to be any point inviting something into the body that has a name like "perfluorocarbon resin." It's too much of a risk.

The Best Choice: Heavy Stainless Steel

Today's most durable cookware also boasts the lowest upkeep. Stainless-steel cookware should be solid and have a vacuum-sealed lid. Thin stainless steel will boil water but will not form the necessary vacuum seal to properly cook food for the best nutritional value. Stainless steel by itself is a poor conductor of heat, requiring high cooking temperatures and more water than usual, which are two conditions to be avoided in cooking.

The most scientific cooking method, the one that retains the most food nutrients, uses heavy stainless-steel, waterless cookware.

This cookware has an outer and an inner surface of pure stainless steel with a core of hard carbon steel between, which acts as a heat conductor and control and forms a vacuum. The weight is important for heat retention. Intended for stovetop use, it is more expensive than other utensils but is a lifetime investment in good health.

Pressure Cookers

Once very popular, pressure cookers are not seen much anymore. Although it saves time, pressure cooking is not the best way to prepare food, because the high-heat conditions it requires will remove the valuable nutrients in the food. Since minerals and vitamins are impaired, the electromagnetic energies are dissipated. If a pressure cooker is used, it should be made of stainless steel and limited to uses like canning foods, for which it is the safest method.

Testing for the Best Baking Equipment

The first choice for cookie sheets, pie tins, muffin tins, bread pans, and cake pans is heavy dairy tin. It conducts heat evenly and wears well.

Unfortunately, distinguishing dairy tin from aluminum is hard. Here is a way to test: a magnet will not cling to aluminum, but it *will* cling to tin. Also, by the way, a magnet will not cling to thin stainless steel, but it *will* cling when the steel contains a nickel or iron alloy, which heavy stainless steel does.

Microwave Ovens

A microwave oven plays an important role in the kitchen laboratory. Many people consider it somehow "nutritionally incorrect" to use a microwave. However, Dr. Parcells found that bread cooked in a conventional oven retained far less of its original nutrient value than microwaved bread. Bread baked in the microwave oven, on the other hand, actually increased in nutrient energy.

Microwave ovens cook food *from the inside out;* conventional oven methods cook from the outside in. That is the simple difference, and it matters in nutrition.

The Beauty of Proper Utensils

The kitchen chemist should choose cooking utensils for their practical value. So many people choose tools to cook with based on how they look—the poorest of reasons for keeping utensils around the kitchen. Besides, there is a certain innate beauty in a good tool that helps provide good health.

KITCHEN SANITATION AND TOTAL HEALTH

Kitchen sanitation is one of the most neglected subjects in modern living. Much suffering could be prevented if a few elementary rules of sanitation were carried out in the everyday preparation and care of food. Many colds, flus, and other contagious diseases spread throughout a family. These could be prevented if dishes, table service, and drinking glasses were always properly cleaned.

A separate cloth ought to be kept at hand for cleaning the kitchen sink, because a great many bacteria gather around the water drain leading to the sewer. Also, it's a good idea to have a bottle of Clorox® bleach near the sink; pour a few drops around the drain and allow them to remain there after all dishwashing is finished.

A cracked dish is an open door to infection. Care should be

taken to throw out any dishes that are cracked. Harmful bacteria form in the cracks of serving dishes, plates, and cups. When hot food is placed in these containers, the bacteria from the cracks enter the food.

Handling Foods

It's imperative to wash one's hands after handling meat, poultry, or fish. Each type of animal food may carry bacteria peculiar to its own kind. Beef may harbor brucella; chicken or other fowl, salmonella; fish, helminths and liver flukes; pork, trichina. The presence of these pathogenic organisms may so affect their hosts, our food, that the food is rendered unfit for human consumption. If it is eaten, it can produce serious maladies not easily recognized by accompanying symptoms.

Usually the heat of cooking dissipates or destroys such potentially harmful parasites. However, when meats are handled during preparation the parasites or their eggs may cling to utensils or to the hands and be transferred to other parts of the body or other foods. Here again, rinsing hands in a pan of water containing a few drops of Clorox® bleach (about 10 drops to 1 gallon of water) will ensure reasonable safety. This is especially important when handling poultry and pork.

FOOD MYTHS AND TRUTHS

Much of our recent inadequate knowledge about foods, passed down from one generation to another in an oral tradition of misinformation, seems to cluster around a few very common foods.

Eating Meat

Can meat be part of a healthy eating plan? You bet it can! Dr. Parcells believed that meat is an excellent source of protein, and she included it in many of the nutrition regimes she devised for her clients.

The simple logic she used was that we ourselves are land animals. Meats of all kinds, eaten in moderation, will enhance health.

Believe it or not, she was less enthusiastic about fish, which she regarded as a sea animal and therefore too different in natural chemical makeup to contribute in an essential way to human health. She did make one exception, however, and that was freshwater fish; one of her favorite dishes was a lightly poached Rocky Mountain trout on a bed of steamed, leafy green vegetables.

Many people today are turning away from meat, especially red meat, in favor of chicken and turkey. They are doing so on political or ethical grounds—and that needs to be respected. But there is no specifically nutritional reason to avoid eating meat in moderation. In fact, it can only help build health.

A word of caution, however. All meats, including beef, pork, chicken, turkey, and meat from other animals, are now routinely clogged with toxins of all kinds—growth hormones, antibiotics, and an incredible array of other junk like pesticides, commercial fertilizers, and carbon monoxide. *It's important to clean all meats in the Parcells Oxygen Soak before cooking and eating.* (See Step Three.) Once clean, meat can increase your energy, stamina, and immunity to disease.

Enjoy that steak—but keep it lean and on the small side, clean it before cooking and eating, and, above all, combine it properly with other foods for optimum assimilation.

Sugar

White sugar is made from sugar beets or sugarcane. The plant material is first crushed and pressed several times to extract the juice. The juice is then mixed with lime and put through evaporators and vacuum-boilers. It first turns into a thick syrup and then into a combination of sugar crystals and molasses. A centrifuge is used to take off the molasses, leaving behind brown sugar crystals. Brown sugar is then refined even further; it is dissolved, treated, bleached, filtered, and recrystallized to yield white sugar.

It shouldn't need to be pointed out that a substance manufactured this way is quite remote from its natural state. There is so little nutritional value in white sugar that it is hardly worth speaking about. At each stage of the refining process valuable nutritional elements, vitamins, and minerals are left behind—in the pulp, which is fed to animals, in the molasses, even in what is filtered out of brown sugar to make it white. What we get, white sugar in its final state, has none of the protective elements needed for its proper digestion and use by the body, and it operates as an addictive substance.

Other Sweeteners

Compare white sugar, as a sweetener, to pure, natural honey, which is processed and manufactured by bees in nature with an absolute minimum of technological fussing between the bee and our morning toast.

Brown sugar, although partially processed, is also an alternative to white sugar. Brown sugar still retains some of the natural enzymes necessary for utilizing sugar in the body.

Still another way to sweeten foods is by using the natural sugars in, say, fruit or milk.

Artificial sweeteners are, by definition, not natural. An artificial sweetener, like anything artificial, is an element contrary to the body's natural chemistry and therefore should be avoided. Using artificial sweeteners is akin to using drugs: they are not naturally occurring chemicals. The body will not burn them, so they are stored in the system, waiting to cause trouble at some future time. It should come as no surprise that artificial sweeteners have also been implicated in food allergies.

Salt

On the list of items in the national diet that we are told to avoid, salt is near the top. But what task does salt perform in the body? Is salt harmful, or is it necessary to good health?

Every cell in our bodies floats in a saline, which is to say a salt-based, solution. The main purpose of salt is to govern the sugar balance in the blood. It also controls the function of the adrenal gland, which in turn controls the sugar balance in the body.

With salt, it is best to think in terms of moderation, not elimination.

Dr. Parcells handled many cases where she recommended the simple use of salt and the person's health improved dramatically. One man came to her Los Angeles office for help. He was more than six feet tall and was at that point a walking skeleton. His stomach had been partly removed, and after that every time he touched sugar or any sweet, it would set up a dysentery that would completely dehydrate him.

Drugs had been prescribed for him, mostly sedatives, which he had taken without relief. Diets had also been assigned, eliminating most of his food. Far from providing a remedy, the diets had made the problem worse.

As Dr. Parcells listened to the man's story, her mind went into the kitchen. Recalling the principles of kitchen chemistry, she thought of the cooking rule, "If anything is too sweet, use salt to correct it; if it is too salty, use a sweetener to correct it."

Here was a similar case: sweetness in any form set up a severe dehydration. As she reviewed the principle in her mind, she walked into the kitchen and prepared a drink of salt water. She took it into the office and had the man drink it while he was sitting there.

Within ten minutes he was a different person. He was more vital, more energetic, happier. His pain was entirely gone. In fact, his entire body was functioning normally.

She suggested he take some salt in water about fifteen minutes before each meal, three times a day. He did, and he never had another problem with sugar intake. The man got back to work and went on to create a successful business, all the time enjoying normal weight and vitality.

Dr. Parcells used to like to relate this story because it went to the heart of her theory of kitchen chemistry. All the drugs and diets did nothing but aggravate and deepen this man's health problems. But the application of something simple using a law of nature changed his whole life—as it had changed hers so many years before.

We appear to be a nation of hypertensive cases. More than twenty-seven million people in our country are said to have blood pressure above what is considered normal. The fourth top drug prescribed in the United States for all disorders is an antihypertensive diuretic (the top three are, of course, antibiotics). Authorities make the flat claim that salt causes the retention of fluid, which contributes to hypertension, but many other factors could be responsible for the problem.

Salt is necessary in the chemistry of the cell. Manufactured versions of salt are not nearly as good for health as sea salt. The Parcells Method recommends using sea salt exclusively, because it contains all the minerals related to water—and water is what salt regulates in the body. The water of the sea, evaporated, is in fact very much like the fluid in our cells and our lymphatic systems.

Iodized salt is manufactured salt with iodine added. This is not a good chemical combination. If additional iodine is needed in the diet, obtain it naturally in other foods; kelp and other sea vegetables, for instance, are rich in iodine.

> *Looking at the claims of modern nutritionists regarding the use of salt, I go back in my memory many years, to when I was a young woman working as a wrangler on a big cattle ranch in the West. We drove cattle up to the high meadows in midsummer for a change of pasture. We always took a load of salt with us, and that was deposited near where the cattle went for water. If the cattle were short of salt during the feeding season, they wouldn't shed, their joints would stiffen and swell—they would be found dead.*
>
> *Salt is essential to all life—as important to human bodies as it is to the bodies of animals.*
>
> Dr. Hazel Parcells

Pepper

The other condiment that usually finds a permanent place at our table is black pepper. Black pepper is recommended for sound nutrition, but only if it is ground from the peppercorn at the time of eating. The oil in black pepper becomes rancid upon exposure to air and can create a digestive problem in a very short time. When it is freshly ground, it is actually an aid to digestion.

On this subject, it's good to keep in mind that the oil in *any* seed will become toxic about thirty minutes after it is released from the shell of the seed. When buying seed spices, such as cumin, mustard, coriander, fennel, anise, and so on, the best rule is to purchase them in their whole state and grind them fresh at home in a spice mill or with a mortar and pestle. Home grinding of spices is not only much more healthy, but it enhances flavors of foods to a much greater degree.

One of the most outstanding natural stimulants and healers in the spice cabinet is cayenne pepper. Dr. Parcells used it in scores of applications as a healing agent. It is a considerable aid to the digestive system. In cases of severe bleeding, cayenne pepper, when applied directly to the wound in the form of a poultice, will stop the flow of blood and will go on to help heal the wound. With any wound where inflammation and a lack of healing are in evidence, cayenne pepper will help to clear up the situation.

To people who are cold all the time, a capsule of cayenne pepper, taken especially before retiring, will warm the entire body from within. Cayenne pepper restores warmth by gently stimulating the whole system. Dr. Parcells used to advise the sprinkling of a little cayenne pepper in the socks for people whose feet are always cold; she had great success with this commonsense approach to increasing body heat.

Many healing properties await our attention in ordinary, natural foods. Not everyone is trained in the chemistry of the marvelous healing capabilities of familiar foodstuffs. But the wonderful thing about using common foods we find in the kitchen cabinet for self-healing is that we can experiment, within reason, to see what works and what doesn't without running a health risk.

> *When Dr. Parcells recommended something quite ordinary to people for their ailments—a glass of water with some apple cider vinegar at the first hint of a cold, for instance, or warm water with a pinch of baking soda for indigestion—she often met with raised eyebrows.*
>
> *That's when she told them, "Well, this may not help you— we won't know until you take it. But it surely won't hurt you."*

All About Fats

When it comes to food fact and food myth, no other food type is more controversial than fat.

Probably the biggest nutritional fad of the past few years has been the concern about dietary fats. Advertisers have pushed onto a nutritionally naive public the notion that fats in the diet, no matter what their nature, will result in all kinds of health hazards from obesity to hypertension, heart disease, strokes, and just about any other ailment in the long catalog of modern bodily disorders.

The truth is, fats have a tremendous value to total health, and throwing them out of the diet entirely, as some so-called nutritional authorities have recommended, is downright irresponsible. We need to go beyond the claims of mass manufacturers of food and their promotional departments to learn the real purpose of fats. Fats have an essential function in the body as a builder. Fatty acids compose some 60 percent of the brain.

The liver is the only organ in the body that makes chemical changes in the fat chain. Fats from any source—from meat to seeds —go to the liver to be broken down and processed. Liver health is an intrinsic part of the fat scenario. A healthy liver will transform fats into usable body material and energy; an unhealthy liver will have trouble metabolizing fats and will be compromised further in its attempts to do so efficiently. Introduction of the right fats will enhance the operation of the liver and of all the other organs in the system.

Fat functions as the protective coating for the spinal cord and eyes—and that is about as significant a role as one single substance can play in the body. Fat produces the covering and protection for the entire nervous system. It is deposited under the third layer of skin to hold in the moisture and chemicals for the skin. Fat operates in the body as its protective element and therefore it is enormously valuable.

> *The residents of Crete eat more fat than any other people. About 45 percent of their calories come from fat, and a whopping 33 percent of their calories come from olive oil. It should follow that Cretans have more heart disease and die earlier. Wrong, Crete is one of the anomalies on the heart disease–fat consumption charts. In fact, the population of Crete has one of the world's lowest rates of heart disease and cancer. Scientists trying to ferret out the "longevity factor" often settle on olive oil. In Crete the olive oil flows like wine. Crete consumes more olive oil per person than any other nation. Not far behind are Italians, Greeks, and others in the Mediterranean area.*
>
> Jean Carper, in *The Food Pharmacy,* 1988

OLIVE OIL   Olive oil is one of the most versatile ingredients in the daily diet. In her home, Dr. Parcells kept extra pure virgin olive oil on the table at every meal. She recommended it for cooking, for baking, for salads. It makes an excellent emollient for the skin. Studies have shown it to be helpful in reducing the level of cholesterol in the blood. She would have no other oil around.

High temperatures destroy the most vital nutrients in oils (as they do in every other type of food). When buying olive oil, go for "extra pure virgin"—the first pressing of the olives—and "cold pressed," which does not use nutrient-destroying heat to extract the oil.

BUTTER   What about butter? The good news is that butter is *good* for us! Who says healthy eating isn't delicious?

Butter contains all the essential oils needed by the body, especially in the nervous system. We receive a great health benefit from using it in moderation. Butter is a natural fat, and wherever fats are required in body function, it is used quite well.

Cream, from which butter is made, is a highly usable natural element, because it is a part of what has already been produced and transformed through the natural processes of the animal and already contains many of the essential oils and oil-soluble vitamins necessary for good body function. Genuine butter is made from cream and contains all the elements present in cream, and more.

When natural fats like butter are removed from our daily diet and totally artificial, manufactured items are substituted, our circulation undergoes a complete change—and cholesterol begins to develop and build up in the bloodstream.

In her five years of intensive research into the components of blood in the 1950s—just when margarine was coming into prominence as a butter substitute—Dr. Parcells saw dramatic changes in liver function in the subjects she studied. Where there had been no previous health difficulties, cholesterol had begun to block the entire circulatory system, leading to damage in the heart valves. At that time, the blame for disorders stemming from the problem was placed on the heart—*a perfect example of how treating only symptoms can never bring about a true healing.* Suddenly, we began to hear a great deal of talk about open-heart operations and replacements of hearts damaged beyond repair.

Artificially produced fats like margarine are taken to the liver for processing—just as natural fats are—but the liver is unable to process the manufactured products for use by the body. The liver is designed to process only forms of natural fats. Not knowing what to do with the artificial substances, the liver simply stores them away until they are picked up by the blood and enter the bloodstream as sticky, heavy, unusable materials. A certain type of cholesterol does have an important part to play in the normal functioning of the blood, but the kind of cholesterol made by accumulated clumps of unused artificial fats is only harmful.

Waste products from artificial fats like margarine eventually reach the valves of the heart, where enormous damage is done. Even before that, they have depressed the function of the liver, which has the job of being the cleaning filter of the system and assigning building work to usable fuel like natural fats.

It's best to use butter in its natural state—that is, not for cooking (heat will diminish its health-giving benefits). A pat of butter on oatmeal in the morning or on brown rice or a potato with the evening meal adds flavor and builds health.

Leave all those manufactured spreads behind on the supermarket shelves. Go instead for pure butter. Use it in moderation, but use it—and don't be afraid that it's going to throw a healthy eating regime off track. It won't. Butter actually contributes to good health.

> *In my laboratory in Los Angeles, I would take a wet drop of blood from clients and place it on a glass slide under a heated microscope. There was the melted fat! It hadn't been absorbed or used by the body; it was there, in the blood, visible in its movement under the heat. When I inquired of those clients what type of fats or oils they used in their homes, the answer always came back, often with tremendous pride, "Why, only margarine!"*
>
> Dr. Hazel Parcells

Dairy Products

Milk is one of the heaviest mucus-forming foods we have. Mucus represents partially digested foods. It forms in the stomach and is transferred to the sinus cavities and nasal passages for elimination from the body.

> *When I was fifteen, I was working on a farm in Colorado. I had just finished my morning chores and was taking the full milk buckets indoors when a group of men rode up on their horses. Their leader had a big mustache and wore spectacles.*
> *"Is that milk fresh, young lady?" he asked.*
> *"The freshest, Mister. I milked ol' Bessie just now."*
> *The man smiled. "Well, I love fresh milk—all by itself. I'll buy some of it from you."*
> *"No need, Mister," I said. "There's plenty. Drink away." I handed him the bucket and a ladle.*

> *He drank one scoop, then another, then another, until he had drunk almost half the bucket. He wiped his mouth with his handkerchief and smiled again. "Ah, Mother Nature—isn't she grand?"*
>
> *After they rode away one of the farmhands came over to me and asked if I knew who the man was.*
>
> *"Some stranger," I said.*
>
> *"Ha! You didn't even recognize him. That's President Teddy Roosevelt."*
>
> Dr. Hazel Parcells
>
> *The brief encounter between the young Hazel Parcells and Theodore Roosevelt took place in 1904. Roosevelt had become president upon the death of William McKinley in 1901 and was running for the presidency that summer, campaigning in the West with veterans of his volunteer cavalry unit, the Rough Riders. He won the presidency and, two years later, signed into law both the Meat Inspection Act and the Pure Food and Drugs Act, the first government legislation to regulate the quality of foods and medicines.*

When we stop to think about the value milk supplies the young for growth and cell building, it is good to remember that a human mother's milk is chemically constituted to provide nourishment and building material for a human animal that probably will weigh from 120 to, say, 220 pounds at maturity; cow's milk has been formulated by nature to support the development of an animal that will weigh perhaps a ton or more. Moreover, cow's milk is rich nourishment for the quick growth of a calf: a calf matures in 2 years, a human matures in 20 years.

Intake of mother's milk should stop when a baby's teeth come in. At that point the infant should begin to eat soft foods such as cooked whole grains. The digestive elements for the heavier material will be supplied by nature.

One of the established dietary rules is to give cow's milk to a growing child. This is a rule that needs to be reexamined. If a child is given milk, it should be between meals or on an empty stomach. Milk does not mix well with other foods, especially other animal proteins. If a child sits down to a meal and, before any food is eaten, drinks a glass of milk, the appetite is satisfied and there is no demand for the good, nutritious food so necessary for health and growth. "Drink your milk" is not a good idea at a meal, unless the milk is properly combined with other foods.

Considering the difference in size between a cow and a human infant, goat's milk might be a better substance for the nourishment of a child; at least a goat is somewhat within the weight range of a human being.

Last, mixing milk from different cows goes against the rules for good digestion. (Avoiding mixing proteins is the first food-combining recommendation above.) The milk on supermarket shelves is mixed, of course, and therefore contains, in each quart or half gallon, different protein structures with different combinations of enzymes, minerals, vitamins, and so on.

NATURAL OVER ARTIFICIAL, FOR GOOD HEALTH

You should be seeing a general rule of nature emerging from all this, and that is, wherever we have a choice between a natural food and an artificial one, we do best to go for the natural. Between the refined and natural sweetener, take the natural; between manufactured salt and evaporated sea salt, take the sea salt; between margarine and butter, by all means take the butter.

These are principles of living with nature—and we will always be more healthy if we follow them.

WHAT YOU CAN DO TODAY FOR BETTER HEALTH

- Combine foods properly. Be creative and enjoy concocting healthy meals according to these simple recommendations: eat only one protein at a meal; eat meat, poultry, and fish separate from dairy products; eat meat, poultry, fish, and dairy products separate from most starches (unless a green leafy vegetable is included).

- Select cooking utensils with great care, and scrupulously avoid aluminum cookware and aluminum foil.

- Be a health sleuth: get to the bottom of food myths—many of them are just that, myths, not truths.

- Design all your eating around natural foods—foods that are "in season," fresh and alive.

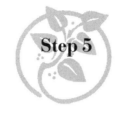

Step 5

CLEAN LIVING

A healthy lifestyle is like a priceless vase that holds beautiful flowers. Without the vase of life-giving water, the most exquisite bouquet of flowers will wilt and die; held within the vase, the flowers will radiate their fragrance and their healing energy to all who encounter them.

DR. HAZEL PARCELLS

THE HOME ENVIRONMENT: AIR AND LIGHT

Late one spring afternoon at Sapello I was working alone at the computer, trying to master a new word-processing program. I had closed the windows and pulled the drapes shut to see the computer screen better.

Suddenly I heard noises behind me, and the room began to lighten. Dr. Parcells was parting the drapes and opening the windows—and muttering something under her breath. I greeted her and asked what she was doing.

"Trying to prevent malnutrition in a writer! Don't you know you need good, clean air and light if you're to be healthy? You need them as much as you need good, clean food. And the house needs air and light for its own health."

I *knew* that, I said to myself.

Home is a special place. It's where we live. The first considerations of health in the home environment are air and light. A home deprived of oxygen is very much like a body deprived of oxygen: it won't live up to its highest potential—in fact, it may smother and die. Without proper attention to light, a home, like our physical self, will languish and lose its sense of vision.

Ventilation is such a basic thing, but we often don't give much thought to the movement of air through the rooms of our home. Air is life, and the movement of air through the home is our home in the process of breathing.

Stale air or air infused with unhealthy smells will have an impact not only on our bodies, but also on the relationships between family members. Tobacco smoke in the air of a home decreases the oxygen content and will lead to health problems over months and years. Smells from accumulated garbage or from pet boxes will bring on depression, cause arguments to break out, and make people irritable. Toxic smells from paint, harsh cleaning agents, glues, or polishes—whether you are redecorating or engaged in some hobby—can affect health.

Today more than ever before, much of our breathing expansions are limited to artificial air—air that has been sprayed with cleaners, air that is filtered and "purified," recycled air from air conditioners—until we have no natural oxygen at all. We need to have expansion if we are going to increase our capacity; when we have nothing but artificial air to breathe from fans and electrical units, the cells in our body are robbed of their proper nourishment.

Good ventilation for health is easy to arrange if we remember to do it. In warm months, keep windows open a bit to allow air to circulate through the home. Even in colder months, it is good to open windows a crack, especially in bedrooms. Sealed-off rooms build up toxicity from stagnation. We *use* the oxygen in our air and expel carbon dioxide. Plants around the home will do the opposite—take in carbon dioxide and release oxygen—so it's a good idea to have house plants: they are effective natural air filters.

A good practice is opening the home in the morning to fresh air. Even during winter months in cold climates, the house can be oxygenated with a brisk rush of new air and the possibility of radon gas accumulations reduced. There are psychological benefits to opening all the doors and windows in the home for a few minutes in the morning: we're greeting the new and establishing our readiness for fresh experiences, challenges, and joys.

Dr. Parcells did five years of research on lighting in the home, because she felt it has a distinct place in healthy living. In looking into the effects of light on biological systems, she found that mice, for instance, developed certain physical abnormalities in reaction to too much or too little light. She went on to learn that all the various devices and types of lights used in home lighting affect people enormously.

Fluorescent light gives off low-grade X rays (which is a health danger) and even affects the visual range negatively. When fluorescent lights are replaced by full-spectrum lights, aberrations in vision disappear. Something else: full-spectrum, or "natural," lighting appears not only to restore and heighten elements of vision, but also improves hearing. As a bonus, the temperaments of the people in the home appear to lighten and brighten.

For full-spectrum lights, check with your local hardware store or health food store. Also, Parcells Center can direct you to the best available full-spectrum light on the market. For prices and more information contact:

Parcells Center
P.O. Box 2129
Santa Fe, NM 87504–2129
1–800–811–6784

Radon, a colorless, odorless, tasteless gas, occurs as a by-product of decaying radium and uranium in rocks and soil.

University of California, Berkeley Wellness Letter, February 1995

[Every year] the radioactive [radon] gas in residences causes about 4,700 lung cancer deaths among nonsmokers, and about 9,700 among smokers.

Journal of the National Cancer Institute, June 7, 1995

Today, of the nation's 150,000 lung cancer deaths each year, public health authorities estimate that almost 10 percent are caused by exposure to radon.

Michael Castleman, "Sleeping Problems," in *Sierra*,
July/August 1993

Radon enters a house through cracks in the foundation, around water and sewer pipes, or in well water. Radon levels are almost always highest in a basement (or first floor, if there is no basement).

Consumer Reports, July 1995

> *When I was doing nutritional counseling in California, I encountered a family with a terrible problem. The family members had usually been compatible with one another, and family life had been rather tranquil. Then it suddenly erupted in irrational behavior and bickering. Seemingly out of nowhere, the daughter had pitted herself against the father; the two young sons were at each other's throats; the parents had begun to shout at each other when they spoke—when they did speak, which wasn't often.*
>
> *I traced the cause to a new streetlight that had been installed outside the home. The large, glaring lamp was sending a brash, irritating light in through all the front windows, disturbing the delicate energy fields of these people.*
>
> *Through a friend who sat on the city council, we were able to have the light removed. In three days, the household returned to normal.*
>
> Dr. Hazel Parcells

Full-Spectrum Light in the Home

Earlier we saw the great benefits to be derived from drinking water purified by exposure to full-spectrum light. By placing a glass gallon jug of tap water under a full-spectrum light for about thirty minutes, we can create water brimming with energy, with a totally different, wonderful taste.

Full-spectrum light performs the same miracle in the air as it does in water. It sheds excellent energy around the room with its light. It improves vision and hearing, and it also seems to improve the mental attitudes of people, allowing them to relax more and to communicate well with each other.

Recent research shows that full-spectrum lights in nursing homes increase the vitality and mental alertness of the residents.

In schools, full-spectrum lights have a calming effect on hyperactive children; learning-disabled children exhibit greater learning ability.

It may sound peculiar, but inferior lighting in the home can create an irritating environment and keep the people who live in it in bondage to a constant state of inner turmoil, which can, in time, become hostility.

Children, particularly, are quite susceptible to the nuances of lighting in the home. Full-spectrum lights installed in their bedrooms, replacing regular incandescent lights, will encourage calm demeanors and cooperative ways.

Television Is Light, Too

Television brings an altogether different kind of light into the home—and it is not a good light. People sit for hours directly exposed to low-level radiation from a cathode-ray tube beamed onto a fluorescent television screen. The rays actually poison the air in the room. Accumulation of these rays in the body over time will damage health, causing a slow erosion of the immune system.

Television also creates a toxic environment in another way. Not only is the technology of television a deterrent to health, but its content, often violent, inhumane, and morally questionable, generates an unhealthy environment in the home. Images are as influential as any of the powerful forces of energy. They are convincing and potent; toxic images can affect us in fundamental ways to the detriment of our health.

Television is especially detrimental to children. It not only interferes with their general physical well-being, but it affects their mental activities and moral attitudes as well. A child exposed to long periods of television viewing matures under the powerfully suggestive guidance of television programming—and we know too well the nature of that content, which is driven by commercial motivations to appeal to the lowest aspirations in people.

Television viewing, being essentially a passive activity—if it can be called an activity at all—acts as a depressant on the body and the mind. It's not difficult to connect the pervasiveness of television viewing in our culture and the pandemic of depression under which many people live, as if yoked to unending misery.

Anything depressive is toxic. The deeper our culture sinks into depression, the more toxic our cultural environment becomes. People have less control over their lives, because living in a depressed state lowers physical energy and clouds judgment. Depressed people operate in an alkaline field, with diminished immune system function, and so are open to every variety of physical, psychological, and emotional affliction.

We may not think of television as contributing to the ill health of an increasingly sickness-prone culture, but it most certainly does. When we consider all the things surrounding us in our home environment, television is one of the most visible and most powerful. Being aware of its presence, in the same way we are aware of light, sound, air, and all the other influences on our physical senses, can encourage us to treat it with extreme caution in our attempts to create an atmosphere of healing in the home.

Average Television Viewing Time per Week in 1995

17 hours and 47 minutes

(Source: Nielsen Media Research)

Hours of Television Viewing Time per Person in 1993

1,429 hours

(Source: World Almanac, 1996)

Percentage of U.S. Homes with Television

1970	95.3 %
1980	97.9 %
1990	98.2 %

(*Source:* World Almanac, *1996*)

Violence predominates on television, often including large numbers of violent interactions per program. . . . Overall, the study finds that premium cable channels like HBO and Showtime are the most violent, with 85 percent of their programming including some violence, followed by basic cable channels with 59 percent, and independent television shows with 55 percent.

Report by Mediascope, in the *New York Times*, February 7, 1996

It is estimated that preschoolers view approximately 27 to 28 hours of television per week, children six to 11 years of age view approximately 23 to 24 hours per week, and teenagers watch approximately 21 to 22 hours per week. By the time of high-school graduation, the average child has spent a total of 15,000 to 18,000 hours in front of the television (compared with 12,000 hours spent attending school).

"Children and Television," in *American Family Physician*, 1994

HEALTH IN THE BEDROOM

Dr. Parcells had a client who had been suffering from insomnia for years. Finding no nutritional cause for the woman's problem, she asked about her bedroom and was told that it was decorated, and had been for years, in a jungle motif—imitation zebra-skin sheets and drapes, wall hangings of monkeys in trees, and all of it set against a background of tropical colors of red-orange and bright green.

"There's your problem," Dr. Parcells said. "You're trying to get some sleep while your bedroom is engaged in monkey business all night!"

If you want a good night's sleep, be certain in the first place that your bedroom has colors on the walls conducive to rest. Pale, pastel pinks or blues or greens are the best. And those colors should extend to window coverings and other decorations in the bedroom.

Sheets, pillowcases, anything that touches the skin should be as natural as possible—not painted with designs or dyed with artificial colors.

Mirrors should be functional, not decorative. Too many mirrors create a cacophony of energy in the bedroom, with images and vibrations bouncing off one another like balls in a pinball machine. Mirrored walls can be disorienting on the unconscious level, particularly when two mirrors are hung across from each other on opposite walls.

Another consideration in the bedroom, as in all the rooms of the home, is the placement of furniture and other items. A chair or table or chest of drawers set in the wrong place can block the energy of the room. If possible, the bed should be placed on the east-west axis, so that the head of the bed faces east, the rising sun.

The best way to sense for obstructions in the bedroom, as in any room, is to slowly walk into and around it with awareness, making certain the path around the room is unencumbered. The circulation of energy, like the circulation of air, is important and health-promoting.

Home Accident Deaths 1950–1994

Year	Total	From solid or liquid poison
1950	29,000	1,300
1960	28,000	1,350
1970	27,000	3,000
1980	22,800	2,500
1990	21,500	4,000
1991	22,100	4,500
1992	24,000	4,800
1993	26,100	5,600
1994	26,700	6,400

(Source: National Safety Council)

The bathroom is the second most dangerous room in the house, the site of about 200,000 injuries a year. . . .

The kitchen is one of the most dangerous rooms in any household, with falls, fires, poisoning, cuts, and electrical shocks leading the list of potential accidents.

The Columbia University College of Physicians and Surgeons Complete Home Medical Guide, 2d ed., 1989

PAYING ATTENTION TO
THE BATHROOM

You've read stories about movie stars and opera stars who have held court in their bathrooms—and kings and queens who literally held court there.

The bathroom is for elimination and for cleaning and grooming. It's a vital place in the home, as those functions are vital to life. A bathroom's size is usually an indication of the importance placed on the eliminative and cleaning activities—too small in most homes. The ideal bathroom should be large enough to move around in and should have separate areas for elimination, body cleaning, and bathing, particularly therapeutic bathing.

Plants are good in the bathroom, especially medicinal plants like aloe vera. They filter the air, add oxygen to it, and give off a pleasant life-energy. Moisture from showering and bathing will feed them and keep them in good health.

Function should be considered over fussy decoration. Avoid carpeting on the floor, since it will harbor all kinds of unwanted bacteria that can end up being a health hazard. Material coverings that disguise toilets and try to make them pretty are traps for germs and fungi and encourage transmission of contagious illnesses.

The best color for the bathroom is white—the color of purity and cleanliness. Even towels and washcloths are better white; it's harder to tell when dark-colored towels or towels with bold patterns are soiled. Towels should be changed frequently. It goes without saying, of course, that if two or more people are using the same bathroom, each should have a different towel and washcloth.

A window in a bathroom is a definite plus: not only will needed light come in from it, but eliminative energy will be released from the home through it.

Finally, a word about general cleanliness in the bathroom. Soaps and shampoos should be chosen for their mild cleaning attributes, not for their perfumed scents. The harsh chemicals in some soaps dry the skin and open it to be host to all kinds of parasitical bacteria. Experiment with natural, unscented soaps and shampoos and brands that contain olive oil or aloe vera, both of which will soothe the skin and scalp. Try two tablespoons of olive oil in a hot tub for relaxation and the care of dry skin.

Dry brushing of the body and the hair will promote health by stimulating the skin and opening the pores for detoxification. Take care that the brush or loofah is not harsh or abrasive—with dry brushing, a little goes a long way. It's always best to brush before showering or bathing, so the toxins released from the skin can be washed away.

The best dry brushing technique is to brush upward, starting with the soles of the feet—up the legs and torso to the chest, up the back, up around the shoulders, and down to the chest, where the nerve centers of the lymphatic system reside. A dry brush should be kept dry at all times to keep harmful bacteria from lodging in it.

Bleach will help keep sink, tub drains, and toilets free of bacteria—a few drops every couple of days will do. Half a cup of bleach in the toilet bowl once a week for fifteen minutes will keep the bowl clean and fresh smelling—it's better than any of the "specialized" toilet bowl cleaners on the market. A few small containers of baking soda set around the bathroom will absorb odors much better than scented chemical "air purifiers" or sprays—which should not be used in any case, particularly in a bathroom without an open window.

THE KITCHEN— HEART OF THE HOME

Years ago people used to spend more time in the kitchen than in any other room of the house. That was at a time when the preparation of food was not only more time-consuming, but much more enjoyable as well. Still, we love to go into the kitchen to see what's happening there, to meet other family members, to talk, and to linger.

Full-spectrum lighting here, as everywhere in the home, generates positive energy fields that enhance life function. Colors in the kitchen need to be considered carefully. White is always good, and any of the soft pastel shades can compliment the needs of the work to be done there. The kitchen is the laboratory of life, remember—the greatest chemical laboratory in the world, except the laboratory of our own body.

The color yellow is a digestive aid. Pale lemon yellow on walls and window coverings where food is prepared and eaten will prepare the body for digestion and encourage more thorough assimilation. The color should be selected with care, though; a yellow too dark or harsh might have an irritating effect. Go for subtle, pastel shades.

Color in the kitchen also extends to the color of food, of course. Every color has a chemical value because every color is essentially a chemical. Chemical components of foods contribute to their crucial acid-alkaline balance. The color of food stimulates growth factors in the body and reinforces the immune system.

It's important to be aware of food colors when planning meals. A selection of colors makes an attractive plate; beyond the appearance, though, a nutritional principle is at work—the balance of colors is also the balance of food chemistry. If you are cooking with colors, you are cooking with total health in mind.

UNCLUTTER THE CLUTTER

We've all heard about people who pass on and leave houses filled to the brim with huge inventories of bric-a-brac, stacks of old magazines and newspapers, and accumulations of "stuff" from years past. Newcomers going into such spaces always report their amazement that so many things could be crammed into so little space.

"Things" not only clutter up the living space of a home, they also are barriers to the flow of energy. Part of good health is sensing when enough is enough and occasionally throwing out the encrustations of the past so the freshness of the new can come in. Keeping energy obstructions down to a minimum will bring health to a home and to all who live in it.

HOW ABOUT THE WORKPLACE?

In the 1980 film *Nine to Five*, three women turn a cold, lifeless, and rigid workplace into a warm, life-promoting, and flexible home away from home. They create a humane schedule that allows employees to get their work done *and* live their lives fully; a day-care center is moved into the conference room; windows are put in, opening dead wall space; plants are everywhere. The result is that three times as much work is accomplished, making three times as much profit for the company.

The workplace can be transformed into a health place. It can be done, and it *should* be done. With luck, if you undertake to humanize your workplace, you won't have to go to the extremes the movie characters went to—stringing up the boss—to accomplish the task.

All the recommendations here about fostering health in the home can also be applied to the workplace. Air and light are at the top of the list of matters to attend to. If your workplace is not ventilated properly, bringing in fresh air and letting out old and used air, you may have to get to work on this before you get to work on your work.

Full-spectrum lighting will improve vision and hearing—and it will also, therefore, improve productivity (a card to play if you need to negotiate with a reluctant or skeptical boss).

Windows are essential to the space where work is done. They bring in light and air from the outside and allow the release of the stale, used air; they are the eyes and lungs of the workplace. In the absence of windows, be aware of air flows through the space, and, by all means, install full-spectrum lighting to take the place of natural light.

If you work around electronic machines, you need to be aware of radiation generated and emitted by them. Even the most advanced-looking technology is giving off rays that can be harmful to health. Look into getting special radiation-blocking screens to put over computer terminals. If you sit at a computer during most of your work day, remember to take a therapeutic bath once a week to release the effects of dangerous radiation from your body. (See Step Two for specific directions.)

Plants are a tremendous help to a healthy workplace. However, make certain they are the right plants for the space, that they can be in touch with natural light, if possible (or with full-spectrum light, if not), and that they are well cared for. Nothing is as damaging to morale on the unconscious level as seeing and working around a plant that is neglected, has yellowing leaves, looks fatigued, and is headed toward death. We pick up the plant's distress and, somewhere in our minds, translate it to our own physical condition. A wilted, dried-out, lifeless plant in the workplace can make workers ill.

It's a good idea for health purposes not to eat in the same place where work is done. Our bodies pick up signals about places. Digestion will be better when you eat in a space assigned for eating.

Having lunch at the desk or the worktable introduces confusion on a subtle level, and that confusion can have an impact on health.

It should go without saying that being at work doesn't mean that we're on vacation from healthy living habits. The challenge is to bring the sense of our healthy home environment into the workplace, to extend the feelings of comfort, pleasure, and the promotion of true nourishment from the place where we live to the place where we work. Work is part of our lives—sometimes a very large part—and therefore health in it deserves the same attention we give to health in the home.

Hours the Average American Spends in the Workplace

during a year	about 2,000
during a lifetime	about 86,000

Number of Fatal Occupational Injuries in 1994

6,588

(Source: Bureau of Labor Statistics, U.S. Department of Labor)

FEELING GOOD BY MOVING AROUND: EXERCISE

Exercise has as important a function in good health as the food we use to support our bodies. Physical activity allows us to maintain a normal response to the demands put upon the muscle structure, which accommodates our power to act under demand.

Fortunately, we are living at a time when the value of exercise is well known. Fitness has been on the rise in the national consciousness the past few years. It is an enormous aid to good health.

Individuals differ in how much exercise they need for proper body operation and optimum health. Many facets of the person need to be taken into account, for example, body type, muscular makeup, glandular constitution, and bone structure. All aspects are important, because exercise has an impact on each area.

In the world of a hundred years ago, exercise was based on the demands of everyday life. People walked a great deal. Most jobs, performed without the benefit of the many machines we have today, required more sheer physical labor. People's intake of food was different—food was "whole" and not affected by drugs, additives, depressants, or false stimuli. They were using the minerals in foods in their natural state and in their natural balance.

Walking was then, and is now, very important, except that today when we walk outdoors we are exposed to an environmental situation much different from the one a century ago. Now the air contains less oxygen—and more carbon monoxide. It should tell us something that birds are now flying at higher altitudes, and even then are dropping out of the sky on their flights. For a full, chilling account of the effects of oxygen depletion in the atmosphere, read Rachel Carson's *Silent Spring*, if you haven't already—a book written in 1962 that has as much relevance now as it did then, perhaps even more.

For walking out in the open, select an environment where there is as little traffic as possible and no industrial manufacturing activity. Walking in a contaminated atmosphere can be counterproductive, which is to say that instead of helping us stay healthy, it can cause us to be ill. Walking in nature is the best. If you live in an urban area, go out to the country, far away from the noise and pollution of the city, to a place where plants and trees are furnishing fresh oxygen, where the sun is shining and you can see and hear the gentle movements of nature. If you can't retreat to the country, find something in the city that has the appearance of the country—a park with trees, or even a football or soccer field. Smell the grass: it's brimming with life!

Stretching and bending are good exercises. Massage and exercises such as yoga help to find the stagnant places that retard muscle development. It's good to exercise moderately every day, particularly if your work keeps you in a seated position most of the time.

At the turn of the last century, exercise was a necessity of life. It was demonstrated rather than talked about. A woman doing housework in those days got all the stretching, bending, moving exercise she needed, changing and enhancing the energy flow in her body by natural means. A man lifted, strained, pulled, pushed, and climbed; it was all in a day's work, and all beneficial to health.

Breathing is a part of both exercise and rest. It is a good practice for health to breathe consciously, deeply, and slowly—from the stomach. Hold the breath in, then let it out, and feel the sense of well-being that comes over you.

RESTING: PART OF GOOD HEALTH

Rest is frequently overlooked as a source of good health. Actually it is a very influential factor in maintaining well-being. Relaxing and resting, both mentally and physically, support the demands of the body and maintain the effectiveness of the immune system.

Night rest, of course, is most significant, because it completes a day's cycle. At the end of the day the body is at the point of being spent. Through the relaxation of all its parts—and the all-important deep breathing that accompanies sleep—the body recovers the full strength of the life force.

We can relax without going into a sleep state, unless the mind is overactive with problems that keep us in an enervated state. Learning how to relax fully is an excellent way to build health.

Many people assume that sleep is a way of getting away from the "busyness" of consciousness. It's true that when we go to sleep our consciousness is stilled; we are in another dimension. But if we're not careful, we can carry stress into sleep. The way to leave stress behind is to put something in its place. If we set our minds to work down an avenue other than worry—a pleasant thought, something positive to build or to do—we can be assured of a restful sleep. Worrying has no real value and interferes with good health. If a matter needs reconsideration, that is not worry—it's just mental management.

Meditation used to be one of those things we assigned to people interested in Eastern religions or eccentrics who had met up with a guru and begun contemplating their navels. But in recent years meditation has entered the mainstream of American life—and none too soon. By nature we are not a reflective culture; we are an active lot. Meditation can bring us more into balance. It gives us the opportunity for a breathing rhythm in our lives—working and resting are like breathing in and out; we need both not only for balance, but for survival.

Many meditation techniques are available to people who want to deepen their experience of life (and enhance their health). The best modes of meditation are the ones that are uncomplicated and do not require any kind of religious underpinnings. Even ten minutes twice a day set aside for meditation and reflection will add greatly to general health.

Note: The Balancing Program in Arizona offers a unique and effective form of quieting the mind at home by concentrating on three universal symbols. To find out more about it, contact:

The Balancing Program
P.O. Box 359
Cortaro, AZ 85652
520–744–3016.

> There are many ways of meditating, but it is important for the beginner to avoid trying to accomplish something beyond his immediate understanding. To meditate successfully and without having disturbing, extraneous thoughts intrude, the mode of contemplative meditation is simple and will lead the student, step by step, into higher forms of meditation.
>
> In contemplative meditation, the student . . . contemplates the sun, moon, stars, and tides, and all growing and living things, remembering that the heavens and the earth are filled with everything of which man has need.
>
> Do not seek harmony or health, or even God. These are not to be found; they already are.
>
> Joel S. Goldsmith, in *Living the Infinite Way*, 1961

HEALTH AND HEARING

Hearing is an essential part of our existence and therefore bears upon our well-being. A high, hard noise is very damaging to the ears. Any loud, compelling noise is difficult on the nervous system. We all know what happens to a cat when it hears a loud noise—it jumps straight up and runs for cover. The central nervous system in humans reacts the same way. Our reaction upon hearing a loud noise is rejection and the physical sensation of wanting to get back to normal as quickly as possible.

If you're living in a situation where you are exposed to high noises, it will affect your health. Some people can train themselves mentally to ignore noise, but the noise is still there, and it makes an impact, through the eardrum, on the entire system.

A note here about hearing aids: the batteries in them are made of aluminum, which is a highly dangerous metal. Hearing aids with aluminum batteries are placed against the eardrum, where they can do untold damage. It is no wonder that people have trouble with their hearing; hearing aids made from or containing aluminum, far from helping the situation, can cause total deafness eventually. Aluminum in hearing aids frequently causes a ringing in the ears (although a ringing in the ears may result from other causes as well).

> *So many times I am asked for the secret of my longevity. I can assure you, there are no secrets. There is only the understanding of nature and the everyday practice of nature's laws.*
>
> Dr. Hazel Parcells, on her 106th birthday

CLEANING TOXIC EMOTIONS

Before leaving the subject of clean living, something should be said about the life of the emotions and how it influences total health.

Eastern philosophies have taken the study of the emotional body to high realms of understanding. In traditional Chinese medicine, for instance, each of the internal organs has a counterpart in the emotional body that, if tended to, extends healing to both the emotional *and* the physical areas of operation and function. If one is angry or resentful, it signals some stress in the liver. Knowing this, one can alleviate the stress by going through both the emotional and the physical doors. The person can take physical measures by cleansing the liver and avoiding foods that an irritated liver hates, like fried foods—*and* release the anger or resentment that has manifested itself in a problematic liver.

The next time you feel an intense flush of anger, try sipping a glass of warm water into which you've squeezed the juice of a fresh lemon. See what happens to the anger. This simple liver cleaner will dissolve much of the anger (although the feelings will have to be handled and released at some point if emotional—and physical— health is to be maintained).

So many of our health problems can be traced to emotional and psychological causes. A simple matter like the gradual loss of hearing can be taken for its physical face value and be treated with all kinds of drugs and devices. Or the sufferer can look deeper: is there something I don't want to hear? Are there people I don't care to hear from? Am I quite happy withdrawing from things and people at this time?

After all, we already have an extensive lexicon of physical ills attached to psychological and emotional issues. We may say that a particular person is "a pain in the neck," that a situation is "a headache," or that individuals are "arm twisting" to get their way, "bellyaching" about something they don't like, or "pulling your leg" to tease.

The serene, happy person is the healthy person. It may take time and effort to reach a state of serenity and happiness; it may take surrender and love—wedded, of course, to good habits of healthy living. But the rewards of working toward emotional health are well worth what it takes on all our many levels.

> *The body, like everything else in life, is a mirror of our inner thoughts and beliefs. The body is always talking to us, if we will only take the time to listen. Every cell within your body responds to every single thought you think and every word you speak.*
>
> Louise L. Hay, in *You Can Heal Your Life,* 1987

WHAT YOU CAN DO TODAY FOR BETTER HEALTH

- Bring fresh air and natural light into your home—the home needs nourishment as much as you do.

- Creatively arrange your home environment according to natural principles, paying attention to the movement of air through the rooms of the home and the quality of light in all areas. Full-spectrum lighting will enhance every room, bringing healing "sunlight" to the place where you live.

- Go ahead and be a crusader for good health: extend the principles of healthy living into the workplace.

- Be aware of the health of the emotions. Much of ill health can be traced back to emotional and psychological blockages. Where emotional "dams" have been set up, take them down for better health.

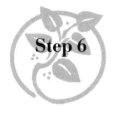

Step 6

HEALING WITH NATURE

Nature, from which we draw all our sustenance, is our ally in self-healing. Over the years of this century we have lost touch with nature and have forgotten many of its healing principles. Bringing nature into our lives again, and embracing it, brings life itself into our experience.

DR. HAZEL PARCELLS

DRUGS AND HEALTH

In 1960, we in the United States spent $27 billion on health care. That figure includes hospital care, physician care, dental and other professional care, home health, drugs and other medical supplies, vision products, nursing home care, and other personal health expenditures, plus "nonpersonal" health expenses for such items as public health, research, and construction of medical facilities.

By 1991, the amount spent on drugs and services had risen to more than $751 billion. Looked at another way, every person in the country spent about $143 on health care in 1960; thirty years later every person spent $2,868.

Our lack of health is costing us dearly. Moreover, our apparent failure to achieve well-being, after all those expenditures, has become an institution in itself: the combination of agencies that treats our increasingly degenerating bodies is referred to as "the health industry."

The bricks and mortar of the health industry are drugs—pills and shots and syrups and sprays prescribed or recommended to alleviate pain. Drugs rarely get to the real cause of a physical malady. They make us feel better temporarily, but they don't get to the core of the problem—nor can they.

"You'll never really get well if you take drugs to do so," Dr. Parcells used to say. "Drugs are a good cover-up, but they never get to the problem, which is a basic imbalance in the organism."

Drugs, like other poisons, increase the pressures to which the body is subjected; removing them allows nature to take over the management of the body. Then, when we're rid of the things that are foreign to nature and therefore foreign to ourselves, our health can improve.

Generally, the Parcells Method opposes the use of drugs of any kind. Drugs either stimulate or depress the body's workings, masking the indications of a disorder. If we simply cover pain, we have lost the opportunity to seek the causes of a health problem. In the process, we have added to the body's burden of difficulties, giving it the further task of dealing with a foreign substance.

A well body doesn't net much profit to those who are seeking a way to earn their living from illness. Except for an occasional accident, I personally have not needed the services of traditional medicine for sixty-five years, so I can't attest to its claims one way or another. I have seen its results in the people who have come to me for advice about self-healing. And much of what I have seen is the damage done by drugs prescribed to treat symptoms of physical discomforts.

Dr. Hazel Parcells

Problems with Antibiotics

Many of medicine's chemical remedies once touted as indisputable cures are becoming less effective in meeting the demands put upon them by physical disorders.

In her lab, Dr. Parcells observed a scenario that went something like this: a disorder was treated by medical science with certain antibiotic drugs; the disorder was taken care of and the person returned to health; then the ailment returned, this time apparently with more force, because the dosage of the drugs had to be increased to handle the problem. Soon she began to see an expansion effect in which ever more powerful dosages of drugs were used for disorders, which seemed to subside for a time, then reappeared.

It was a vicious circle—and, for the people involved, a losing battle.

In *The Coming Plague,* Laurie Garrett reports on the spiraling virulence of *streptococcus.* In 1941, "a dose of 10,000 units of penicillin a day for four days was more than enough to cure strep respiratory infections." Strep A strain was virtually eradicated by penicillins and other common antibiotics, "and it disappeared entirely from the clinical scene. American and European medical students of the 1960s had only picture books to refer to in order to learn what this once-common disease known as scarlet fever was."

By the 1980s strep A had come back in a more powerful form, and by 1992, Miss Garrett says, "the same ailment required 24 million units of penicillin a day, and might, despite such radical treatment, still be lethal."

To put antibiotics in some perspective, look at the development of the king of antibiotics, penicillin. Early in this century it was recognized that plant rootlets secrete highly toxic protective antibacterial substances called "antibiotics." It was Scottish bacteriologist Dr. Alexander Fleming who, in 1928, noticed that no bacteria grew near some *Penicillium notatum* fungus that had accidentally fallen into a preparation of bacteria he was about to throw away. A fungus had knocked out bacteria—and penicillin was born. Note that *anti* means "against," and *biotic* means "life."

In 1940 Howard W. Florey and Ernest Chain developed the first practical application of penicillin. It saved thousands, perhaps millions, of lives. It also spawned scores of other variations of antibiotics—all of which were effective up to a point. But over the half century since their introduction, the ability of antibiotics to kill bacteria has gradually eroded: for protection, the bacteria have been making themselves stronger and fighting back.

> *Penicillin is a specific antibacterial secretion of a fungus. Penicillin was seen as a great miracle and, certainly, when introduced in the middle of World War II, many soldiers' lives were saved because of penicillin. However, there's*

always a price to pay down the road when you do something left-handed with nature.

Dr. Bernard Jensen and Mark Anderson,
in *Empty Harvest,* 1990

Dangers to the Immune System

Antibiotics can compromise health. The introduction of antibiotics into the bloodstream creates havoc with the red blood cells. The basic health profile of a person who has been on an antibiotic program will show heavy residues of antibiotics in the brain, the glands, and the internal organs. Only a thorough cleansing program to remove antibiotic residues from the system will restore good health.

Many antibiotics are alkaline in nature; their habitual use therefore can throw the pH balance of the human system into an alkaline field. Disorders are most often bred in an alkaline field: total alkalinity is one of the physical signs of death.

There may be times when antibiotics are needed, but a health-conscious person will be extremely cautious with their use. Taking antibiotics indiscriminately or too frequently will weaken the immune system. If antibiotics are an absolute necessity, it's best to undertake a complete cleansing program after you've returned to health.

Nature has given our bodies a tremendously sophisticated defense system of their own. Introducing foreign substances like antibiotics to do the work of the body's own healing capabilities is often unnecessary and can delay healing.

Dealing with Antibiotics

- Adopt a lifestyle of good nutrition. Bodies well nourished with clean food and rich with life-energy can usually defend themselves naturally against the invasion of harmful bacteria.

- If a condition has deteriorated to the point where the use of antibiotics is necessary, use them with caution, and do not overuse them.

- After well-being has returned, detoxify the system in a gentle way to clean out the immune-compromising fallout from antibiotics and to restore the body's natural balance. Any of the herbal-based detoxification programs offered at health food stores are appropriate for an internal cleanse of antibiotic residues. The Parcells Detoxification and Rejuvenation Program (Appendix I) is the best internal cleanser, since it detoxifies at the cell level.

> *In this country, obstetricians and gynecologists write 2,645,000 antibiotic prescriptions every week. Internists give out 1,416,000 in the same period. Pediatricians and family physicians lead the way, prescribing over $500 million worth of antibiotics each year to treat just one problem—ear infections in children. Another $500 million-plus is spent on antibiotics to treat other pediatric illness.*
>
> Dr. Michael A. Schmidt, Dr. Lendon H. Smith, and Dr. Keith W. Sehnert, in *Beyond Antibiotics*, 1993
>
> *Antibiotics are powerful medicines that should be reserved for situations that demand them, for instance, when the immune system cannot contain a bacterial infection or when a bacterial*

> *infection establishes itself in a vital organ like the heart, lungs, or brain. Another strong reason to be cautious about overuse of antibiotics is the possibility of selectively breeding new strains of antibiotic-resistant, more virulent bacteria. Even people who are aware of that danger seldom realize that frequent use of antibiotics can lead in the long run to weakened immunity.*
>
> Andrew Weil, M.D., in *Natural Health, Natural Medicine*, 1995

Drugless Weight Management

Recent research reveals that one-third of all Americans carry more weight on their bodies than they should if they are to have optimal health. The same research gives us the depressing news that, in spite of our advanced, sophisticated knowledge of how the body works, the problem is becoming worse.

In discussions of body weight, much is said about obesity, but not much about attaining and remaining in good health. Health is life in balance, which includes the balance of appropriate weight for each and every body.

Weight is about quantity; health is about quality. Our bodies are not machines disconnected from the earth on which we walk. We don't exist somewhere apart from the soil, the water, and the air of this planet. On the contrary, we are an organic part of it. We are the children of mother earth, from whose opulent bosom we take our life and sustenance.

The first fact of nature is that our bodies are made up of minerals. We *are* the earth. We come from the earth and we return to the earth. And while we are living upon the earth, we obtain our nourishment entirely from the earth.

If we are to solve the puzzle of overweight, it's important to look first to the question of true nourishment. We're basically undernourished—not because we don't eat a great quantity of food, but because much of the food we eat has little or no nutritional value.

Early in her long career as a proponent of health, Dr. Parcells responded to people concerned about overweight by designing special eating plans to help them successfully shed pounds. Later, her thinking developed along deeper lines. She concluded that the quality of food, and what the body did with that food, was of paramount importance.

In time she drew up a list of guidelines for people who experienced an imbalance in body weight. Her advice was based on the conviction that a thoroughly nourished person would not be plagued with weight problems.

- Detoxify. Many problems of overweight are due to the accumulations in the body of undigested food. A weight-balancing program begins with detoxification. Cleaning the body on the inside will rid cells of clogged materials, including toxins, that have been slowing down the metabolism. The eight-day Parcells Detoxification and Rejuvenation Program, which cleanses the body at the cell level, is the best way to detoxify (see Appendix I for full details on this program). Other programs are available from health food stores or from your health care professional. Pay particular attention to cleansing of the liver.

- Get nourished. Weight stabilization starts with being truly nourished by the food we eat. Foods in their natural state, fresh, unprocessed, and full of life-energy, will nourish the body in a natural way. Avoid as much as possible any "food" that has been packaged, boxed, treated, manipulated, overprepared, or unnecessarily fussed-over. Go for "whole" foods, i.e., foods in their natural or near-natural state.

- Eat clean, drink clean. Food and drink going into the body should be of the highest quality in terms of life-energy. Anything less will detract from health, acting merely as filler—and will cause problems in weight stabilization as time goes on. The Parcells Method of cleaning will both purify and revitalize food. Drinking water can be cleaned and revitalized by placing it under a full-spectrum light.

- Combine foods properly. Three easy rules will bring about optimum digestion, and thus help in weight stabilization: at the same meal (1) do not mix proteins; (2) do not mix dairy products with other proteins; and (3) do not mix proteins and most starches. Make fresh fruit and vegetables the cornerstone of meals. Include fresh green leafy vegetables in daily meals. If vegetarian plans are best for you, fresh fruit and vegetables, grains, and beans can provide well-balanced meals.

- Be conscious of what you are eating. So much of eating is unconscious, in the sense that we are concentrating on something other than our food and the process of eating when we are putting something into our mouths. Try to avoid eating while driving, watching television, viewing a movie, or talking on the telephone. When it's time to eat, simply eat, with full attention to the act of eating, reflecting all the while on how the food we are taking in is nourishing, revitalizing, and beneficial to the body.

- Exercise. As if we needed to be reminded again, even moderate exercise will enhance health and help to stabilize body weight. Choose exercise that most closely resembles the "working body"—walking, light lifting, running, stretching, bending, climbing. No weight stabilization plan will be successful without daily exercise.

- Understand fullness. To feel "full" is as much an emotional response as it is a physical signal. Emotional issues of being "unfulfilled" may find their way to the dinner table. Holding weight on the body as insulation to keep people or situations away has a fundamental impact on managing weight. Settling emotional issues will aid in settling problems of a weight imbalance.

- Avoid diets. Fad "quick weight loss" diets don't work and actually can be quite damaging to health. For long-lasting weight stabilization, eat small-to-moderate amounts of full-energy food and exercise daily. If the bathroom scale is "the enemy," get rid of it. Remember that weight is about quantity, but health is about quality.

- Accept yourself as you are. At some point, for the good of both physical and emotional health, it is necessary to accept who we are "in the body." If you're doing all you can sincerely to manage body weight and still do not measure up to what you think you're supposed to look like, then maybe your image of yourself needs reexamining. It's difficult to dismiss what our culture presents as the ideal body, but we may have to if we're to retain our mental health. Try to remember, in all serenity and love, that you are who you are—and it's okay.

DAILY EATING SUGGESTIONS FOR WEIGHT MANAGEMENT
Have three or four small meals a day. In the morning, fresh fruit and whole grains. At lunch, a green salad with a small amount of cheese or a serving of meat, poultry, or fish. In the afternoon, vegetables with whole-grain crackers or bread. In the evening, a cooked protein and vegetables.

An example:

Breakfast: Cooked oatmeal with fresh berries

Lunch: Spinach salad with feta cheese, *or*
Fresh vegetable salad with tuna, *or*
Mixed green salad with chicken breast
(small amount of olive oil with lemon juice
or vinegar)
One or two corn tortillas

Dinner: Steamed vegetables, rice, beans, with fresh herb
seasonings, *or*
Leafy green salad, potato, baked or poached
fish, *or*
Steamed greens, polenta, turkey

Between meals, if necessary or desirable, enjoy vegetables or fruit (small quantities of fruit, which is quite sugary).

A reminder about fats: small amounts of real butter and cold-pressed extra virgin olive oil will enhance flavor *and add to health*. Avoid margarine, other vegetable and nut oils, and fats from other animal sources.

Avoid "diet" foods like the plague. Misnamed, they tend to detract from health and, ironically, add to a weight problem.

A good rule to follow: a "food substitute" is not food and therefore will not contribute to nourishment—which is the first requisite for weight stabilization.

> *All high-mineral foods are low in calories, and all high-calorie foods are low in minerals.*
>
> Dr. Hazel Parcells

ESSENTIAL OILS FOR HEALING

One of the newest tools for self-healing with nature is also one of the oldest—maybe the oldest form of medicine in human history. Essential oils are the subtle, volatile liquids distilled from plants, shrubs, flowers, trees, roots, bushes, and seeds. They contain oxygenating properties that transport nutrients to the cells of the body.

Essential oils were known to the ancients, but ways of extracting the oils were forgotten over time, and the medicinal herbs and seeds from which they were taken were used in their gross state instead. Clinical research shows that essential oils help create an environment in the body in which many harmful bacteria, viruses, and fungi cannot live.

They are rubbed directly onto the body, most effectively on the soles of the feet. From there they are absorbed into the lymphatic system, where they bring about marvelous healing. Some of the kinds of essential oils that are available are:

Basil: for intestinal problems, muscle spasms, poor memory, and mental fatigue.

Birch: for relief from bone, joint, and muscle pain associated with arthritis and injury.

Cypress: to restore energy and to help the circulatory system handle edema, cellulitis, varicose veins, and water retention.

Lavender: for universal uses; for skin conditions including burns, psoriasis, and other rashes; helps to create a general feeling of well-being.

Marjoram: to calm the respiratory system and to help relieve muscle aches and pains.

Lemon: to enhance the cleansing of the lymphatic system and to relieve digestive problems.

Spruce: to aid the respiratory, nervous, and glandular systems.

According to the translation of ancient Egyptian hieroglyphics and Chinese manuscripts, priests and physicians were using oils thousands of years before the time of Christ.

There are 188 references to oils in the Bible. Some precious oils, such as frankincense, myrrh, rosemary, hyssop, and spikenard, were used for the anointing and healing of the sick.

Biblical prophets recognized the use of essential oils as a protection against the ravages of disease. The three Wise Men brought the oils of frankincense and myrrh to the Christ child. Scientific research now shows that frankincense oil contains very high immuno-stimulating properties.

Gary Young, in *The Young Living Essential Oils Story,* 1995

The best, purest essential oils on the market are manufactured by Young Living Essential Oils in Utah. Dr. Parcells's last public appearance was as the keynote speaker for the company's annual convention in 1995.

For a catalog of products, contact:

Young Living Essential Oils
250 South Main Street
Payson, UT 84651
1–801–456–5400

COLOR AND HEALING

D r. Parcells met Dr. Francis J. Kolar in Wichita, Kansas, in the early 1940s. Dr. Kolar was in his eighties. His German name sounds like the English word "color," which perfectly describes his life's work: he used color to heal people.

Dr. Kolar had come to this country from Europe and opened a clinic in Wichita. Later he moved to Los Angeles. Dr. Parcells became interested in the effects color had on health and began to work with him.

Back in Europe after World War I, Dr. Kolar had undertaken research into color in Vienna. A dedicated humanitarian, he was looking for ways to help people who had been injured in the war. At the research hospital to which he was attached, he and his staff were performing experiments on laboratory mice. Spinal fluid was drawn from the mice and analyzed. Then half the mice were allowed to go about their normal functions and activities, while the other half were put through a strenuous round of exercise on a treadmill until they were exhausted. Another sample of spinal fluid was taken and examined.

Spectrographic analysis of the spinal fluid of the exhausted mice showed the absence of some of the colors present in the analysis of the fluid of the control mice, which showed a full spectrum of color. It was also found that, upon retesting after the exhausted mice had revived, colors reappeared in the spectrum of their spinal fluid.

The study showed that color accompanied healing, the body's return to a state of wellness and balance. This was the first of many experiments Dr. Kolar performed to plumb the healing properties of color.

For thirteen years Dr. Parcells worked with Dr. Kolar as his nurse and assistant. During that time she became familiar with the direct effect color has on the body and its health. She began to see that people who were ill had "no color," for example, in the gray pallor of their skin or in an analysis of their spinal fluid, which showed lack of color.

It was at that time that Dr. Parcells began to analyze the real meaning of color's connection to health. She found that color is a point of life and a certain sign of it: when a person leaves the body at death, all color also departs the body and rigor mortis sets in. With Dr. Kolar, she went through many different levels of investigation and learned that color is the foundation of our life's energy and the true healing force of the body.

Dr. Parcells used color as a healing agent in all her work. She would shine a light on a person through a colored glass. In some cases she brought an unconscious person back to consciousness with the application of color. She found that shining indigo-colored light over a pregnant woman's pelvic region could enhance the well-being of both mother and fetus; children delivered with the aid of color therapy were born awake and aware and quickly developed far beyond their years.

Whatever method of self-healing is being used, it can always be advanced by using color. Dr. Parcells developed a way of knowing which color is needed and how to apply it. Briefly, her work was based on the principle of finding out which color is missing from the full spectrum of color that indicates health and then applying that color.

Indigo (blue and violet) works remarkably well for insomnia.

Yellow has a stimulating effect on the nervous system, is a digestant, and operates through the intestinal tract in many different and marvelous ways; it also will help correct constipation in people who have had a long history of that complaint.

Lemon yellow is good for the eyes.

Magenta (violet and red) acts as a general gland stimulant.

Orange is an oxygen carrier and acts as a general body normalizer.

Black, which is the absence of color, lowers energy. If you're making a long road trip in an automobile with black upholstery, you'll feel exhausted after an hour of driving. If you habitually wear black clothing, you'll find that your life force and all body functions are lower. Overweight individuals who wear black to appear slim do not reduce their size—they lower their body energy, including their metabolic energy, which impacts negatively on weight management.

Certain shades of pink on walls calm the emotions and lower blood pressure.

Whites and neutral colors in the bedroom assure restful sleep. Conversely, bedrooms with wild colors and patterns disturb sleep and relaxation, memory, even vision and hearing.

Dr. Parcells often said that if all the tools for natural self-healing were taken away from her, save one, she would want that one to be color. The healing power of color is a mystery going back to the sun itself, from which we receive life.

In the future, widespread, wonderful healing work may be done with color. If what Dr. Parcells saw about how it works as a restorer of physical, mental, and emotional well-being is any indication of its promise, that future is bright indeed.

How Color Healing Works

If you've seen a photograph taken by the Kirilian process, you know that the energy that flows out of us is visible with certain lenses and that energy is colored. A Kirilian photograph of a hand shows not only the hand, but the aura of the hand—a halo of light around it—and the aura has colors in it.

A whole science has grown up around the interpretation of the various colors of auras. The colors of the energy in our bodies are related to energy centers called chakras. Aura colors change from moment to moment depending on what is going on in our bodies, that is, what chakras are dominant or throwing off light; each chakra gives off light from its own place on the light spectrum. If we have a Kirilian photograph taken of ourself in an apprehensive state, we will see a red glow around us. Red is the color of the lowest, or first, chakra. It signifies fear, primal instinct, anger, survival, our lower nature. An hour later, with another photograph, we may see a green glow: our energy has moved up through orange and yellow into the fourth chakra, the place of the heart—compassion, understanding, love.

If we were to see ourselves as the energy that we really are, we would see rainbow beings walking around. We glow from within, and that glow is full of color.

The principle of using color for healing is based on the idea that if our health is in a state of imbalance, it will show in the color emanating out of us. When we are deficient in a particular color, we may be able to replace it and regain health.

At some point in the future it might be possible to examine ourselves by actually seeing our color-selves and then applying color to our personal spectrum. Meanwhile, we can approach color healing from the other direction: we can look at the symptom bothering us and add the color that is deficient or missing.

> *Light is the basic component from which all life originates, develops, heals, and evolves. This has been expressed by wise sages and metaphysical texts of the past and present. However, we are about to see a new marriage—between the "intuitive" and the "rational" sciences—a marriage that is bonded by light.*
>
> *There is no such thing as treating the body as a separate collection of "parts" to be fixed when broken. Human beings are the embodiments of light; our troubles and ills result from our inability to take in and use light as a launching pad from which to heal and evolve.*
>
> Jacob Liberman, O.D., Ph.D.,
> in *Light, Medicine of the Future,* 1991
>
> *For further information on Dr. Liberman's book and newsletter, write:*
>
> > *Universal Light Technology*
> > *Box 520*
> > *Carbondale, CO 81623*

How to Use Color for Healing

The simplest way to experiment with color healing on yourself is to hold up a prism made of quartz crystal in sunlight or in front of a full-spectrum light and look through the base of it. Light, which is color, will come into your body through your eyes.

Another way to use color for self-healing is to take a "color bath." Get some cellophane or plastic theatrical gels (which are used to put in front of spotlights to change colors) and hold them up, one at a time, so that sunlight shines on your face through the cellophane or gel. Or simply look through them. This can be done indoors with a full-spectrum light and a lamp rigging for those who are mechanically inclined.

Try looking at the world through a blue gel. See what you feel after a few minutes. You should feel calmer and more relaxed than you did before you began the experiment. If you had been feeling pain before, it should have eased up under the blue light.

Stomach upset will manifest itself in the color-body as a deficiency in the color yellow. Taking a color bath in yellow will add that color to your personal color spectrum, and your stomach should feel better after the color has reentered the body energy.

Still another experiment to perform is one used by Dr. Parcells on herself for many years: make a "color cocktail" by placing a piece of colored glass or a color gel over a glass of distilled water in sunlight or under a full-spectrum light. (No other kind of water will do, because distilled water, unlike other kinds, is a perfect liquid sponge.) Keep the color over the glass of water in the light for ten minutes, then drink the water. You will now have that color in your personal color spectrum. (Note: the water will not change color—it will remain clear, but it will contain the energy of the color.) Check Dr. Parcells's color chart to see which color or colors you might like to use.

Note: The best colored glass to use for this purpose is colored "cathedral glass." Parcells Center makes available a variety of 4-by-4-inch cathedral glass plates. For more information write or phone:

Parcells Center
P.O. Box 2129
Santa Fe, NM 87504–2129
1–800–811–6784

Prism water, or "rainbow water," is made the same way. Place your prism over a glass of distilled water for ten minutes in the sun or under a full-spectrum light. Now the water is full of color. (It still *looks* colorless, however.) When you drink it, you'll have all the colors of the rainbow filling out your personal light spectrum. This is a very high-energy drink. You'll feel reenergized almost immediately.

The beauty of prism water is that you are not treating a specific ailment with a specific color, but giving yourself a flood of color and allowing the full range of colors to fill in the deficiencies, if there are any, in your color-body. High-quality prisms are also available from Parcells Center.

It may sound unfamiliar, even peculiar, but many people believe color therapy is the medicine of the future. Along with equipment for other approaches like sound vibration therapy, hospitals of the next century may be outfitted with color-bath rooms, where patients receive the colors missing from their energy fields that will help them return to health. Some pioneers in color therapy think it was used routinely and with great success in ancient times, but the methodology was forgotten.

Only you can tell if color therapy works for you. If you are in the least bit curious, you might try color baths and see whether they improve the quality of your health. As in all of the recommendations on natural self-healing developed by Dr. Parcells, it may not help—but it surely won't hurt.

> *The Egyptians . . . developed healing temples inside pyramids to take advantage of the universal healing properties of light and color. In Greece, Pythagoras gathered information and taught about the healing light using Egyptian teachings about soul mastery. Heliopolis, the Greek "City of the Sun," had special healing temples in which sunlight was broken down into its different colors to treat various medical conditions.*
>
> Dr. Samuel A. Berne, in *Creating Your Personal Vision: A Mind-Body Guide for Better Eyesight,* 1994
>
> *For information on Dr. Berne's remarkable book, contact him directly at:*
>
> > *The Design Center*
> > *418 Cerrillos Road*
> > *Santa Fe, NM 87501*
> > *505–984–2030*

The Therapeutic Value of Colors

COLORS

Blue

Green

Yellow

Red

Violet

COLOR COMBINATIONS

*"Immunity":**	*red and green*
Indigo:	*blue and violet*
Lemon:	*yellow and green*
Magenta:	*violet and red*
Orange:	*red and yellow*
Purple:	*violet and yellow*
Scarlet:	*red and blue*
Turquoise:	*green and blue*

THERAPEUTIC USES

Blue   *A depressant for motor nerves; remedial for fast pulse, for pain, and for reducing temperature—a pulmonary sedative.*

Green   *An antiseptic; a stimulant to the pituitary gland; builds vitality; works through ductless glands and lymphatics; receptive, it encourages the absorption of medication.*

Yellow   *Acts as a laxative; is a motor nerve stimulant; increases flow of bile; increases stomach and intestinal activity; is a nerve builder; reduces swelling.*

Red   *For vascular contraction (pertaining to blood vessels); an astringent; a hemoglobin builder; a*

*Called such in the color work of Dr. Parcells, because red and green together do not create another distinguishable color of their own.

cerebral (brain) excitant; remedial as a urinary
acidifier; enhances the treatment of tuberculosis;
works through the liver and mucous membranes.

Violet   A cardiac depressant; a motor nerve depressant;
stimulates spleen and the building of white blood
cells; regulates tension of blood vessels; lowers
high blood pressure.

"Immunity"   Used to build up the immune system against
(red and green) infections or bacterial invasions; reduces
fevers; is a protection against any outside
contamination.

Indigo   A sedative; stops hemorrhaging; a depressant for
an overactive thyroid gland; for pain; remedial
for excessive urinary flow and for high blood
pressure; for trauma (shock from accidents and
emotional incidents).

Lemon   An antacid and a laxative; a bone builder; can
be used for brain excitement (for dullness of
memory); especially effective for a sluggish liver.

Magenta   A cardiac stimulant that also aids in bronchial
disorders; a diuretic and urinary alkalinizer
(used to normalize acid urine); aids in dissolv-
ing kidney stones; acts as a general gland stimulant throughout the body.

Orange   A general body normalizer; useful in asthma
or respiration conditions; helpful for spasms; an
aid in digestion and assimilation; relieves ulcers;
dramatically improves thyroid function; is an

oxygen carrier to the lungs; aids the function of all the ductless glands; stimulates vitality.

Purple   *A cardiac (heart) tonic; brings on vascular dilation (pertaining to blood vessels); works through the lymphatics; remedial for poor circulation.*

Scarlet   *A cerebral (brain) stimulant; reduces inflammation; acts as an arterial stimulant; a general healer throughout the body.*

Turquoise   *Increases acid content in the acid/alkaline balance; produces vascular dilation (pertaining to blood vessels); heals mucous membranes; stimulates brain activity.*

WHAT YOU CAN DO TODAY FOR BETTER HEALTH

- Avoid the use of all drugs if possible. Usually they delay true healing by merely masking symptoms.

- Be extremely cautious about taking antibiotics. If it is absolutely necessary that you take them, use them correctly and then undertake a gentle cleansing fast afterward, so that residues will be flushed out of the body.

- Stabilize body weight with good eating habits—avoiding fad or "quick weight loss" diets at all costs. Weight is about quantity; health is about quality.

- Enter the world of color therapy: experiment with color as a self-healing agent. Your body is energy, and energy is colored. Adding color to your personal spectrum can enhance health.

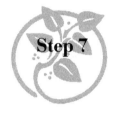

HELPING TO HEAL OTHERS

Every one of us is a healer. Once we have unlocked the secrets of nature and made ourselves free of illness, we need to help heal the people around us. It is a law of healing: doing for others will come around and "do" for us. When we don't move outside ourselves to help others, the circle of self-healing is left open. By helping those near us to apply nature's sublime principles to themselves, we ensure our own better health.

DR. HAZEL PARCELLS

WE ARE ALL HEALERS

It was a rainy Saturday afternoon in early spring at Sapello. The scent of newly invigorated juniper pine was in the air; to the north, misty clouds hugged the foothills of the Rockies; the

Sapello River, a meandering stream swollen now with the melting snow from the mountains, rushed along the outer edge of the property, providing a gentle background hum for returning songbirds.

I made myself a cup of tea and went looking for Dr. Parcells. She was in the lodge house at her desk hunched over a "determination board" with her pendulum. When I asked what she was doing, she kept her eyes on the swinging pendulum for a moment, then looked up.

> *Some are seeing what has been happening in the world and are taking responsibility for themselves and others by adopting styles of healthy living that, only a few years ago, would have seemed single-minded and even radical. My own approach to health is as old as time, but it frequently has been regarded as revolutionary. Still, it is nature's way, and its healing powers are undeniable.*
>
> *In matters of physical well-being, the old way of thinking went something like, "You fix me up. Nothing is required of me." The legacy of that philosophy is with us in the practice of turning our backs on nature and our own common sense in favor of the opinions of the "trained professionals."*
>
> Dr. Hazel Parcells

"You've been complaining of indigestion, so I thought I'd try to find the cause—I mean the *real* cause. And here it is. Not as much activity in the parotid gland as there could be. People like you, who weren't breast-fed as infants, will often have some digestion problems in later life."

I thanked her for taking the time to look into my concern—

then I raced through my memory banks to find out if I had ever mentioned to Dr. Parcells that I was not, in fact, breast-fed as a baby. I hadn't.

"Colostrum is a liquid secreted by the mammary glands immediately after childbirth," she explained. "In the infant, it stimulates the parotid gland, which is tucked in under the ears and chin. If the parotid gland isn't mobilized into action at that time, the proper flow of digestive juices won't be forthcoming. And that diminished operation can follow the person all through life."

In that moment I felt a profound appreciation not only for Dr. Parcells's remarkable thoroughness and dedication to discovering the cause of a health problem, but also for her immense compassion, which had motivated her to forego time she could have spent in a hundred other ways to help me heal myself.

Healing is something we can learn to do for ourselves, but it must never stop there. Its energy of repair and return-to-balance should radiate out from us and touch others, if it's to be truly effective for ourselves.

A principle is at work here that gets at the heart of natural self-healing. It is an understanding of the interconnectedness of all life. We are inseparably part of nature; we are the human layer of the planet, the thinking, reflecting layer of it. Since nature includes every other person, what we do to heal ourselves in a very real sense heals everyone else. The actual act of helping others to health is the acknowledgment of the natural principle of oneness.

This thinking goes against many of our modern ideas about wellness, which place care for the body in the hands of medical "specialists." The truth is that our bodies have been designed by nature as marvelous healing mechanisms—if you don't believe this, see how quickly a cut on your finger will heal, often without leaving a trace, on its own and with no more intervention than keeping the area around the cut clean.

Dr. Parcells predicted a time would come soon when we all would be called upon to take a much more active role in healing ourselves and others—which, in the widest sense, means also healing our ailing planet.

Learning About Healing

What is disease? A breaking down, a breaking apart; the opposite, in other words, of creative energy, which builds. Dr. Parcells believed that there is no need for disease. It's created in confusion, when we surrender to disorganization out of a lack of understanding of natural principles.

The first step on the road to helping ourselves and others to wellness is to learn what the body is and how it works. Most of us learned something about our bodies in school. Classes in personal hygiene and in biology and chemistry gave us some worthwhile information on the mechanics of our bodies. However, that information was probably rather paltry—and school, for many of us, was a long time ago.

If you are sincerely interested in taking charge of your own health and, by extension, helping the people around you to regain and retain their health, do some investigating.

Here are some practical suggestions to foster the emerging healer within you:

• Learn about what the human body is and how it functions.
  Never in history has there been more information available
  on the human organism—whether it's in books, in magazines,
  in newspapers and newsletters, on television, or on the home
  computer (for the computer-literate, the Internet is a great

help in this regard—people are turning to it regularly for answers to health problems).

- Try to sort out information from misinformation. While there are huge amounts of information out there, much of it is contradictory or slanted. The vast majority of "facts" about the body and health are generated by pharmaceutical companies and food supplement manufacturers and marketers. Not all the information is tainted by commercialism, but enough of it is to make us suspicious. Distinguishing between solid information and advertising will clarify the search for truth. With so much sheer volume of information at hand, it's possible to get a second, third, and fourth opinion.

- Observe the workings of your own body. You are, after all, your own healing laboratory. Illness doesn't simply appear like magic; it has a cause. Was it something you ate—or did not eat? Was it the weather, pollen in the air, a cold draft, another person, or physical or mental exhaustion? Was it the way you felt about the world that day? Noting your body's responses to the environment can be the key that unlocks the mysteries of ill health and well-being.

- Be reluctant to name things as diseases. "Cancer" is only a name that medical science has given to certain maladies— so are "arthritis," "lupus," "diabetes," "osteoporosis," and all the other "diseases" in our long catalog of labeled ailments. When illness is named, the brain picks up all the symptoms medical science has associated with it, and suddenly we find ourselves imprisoned in a cage of names and numbers. It's easy to name a feeling of ill health—easier than going looking for the real cause of being out of balance—because in our culture there usually is a specific pill assigned to take care of a specific discomfort. For the true seeker of lasting health, the challenge is to get out from under tags and go looking for causes. In this regard, it would be a good idea to confine reading and research to how your body works and to forget books of symptoms and diseases; highly suggestive, they tend to create what they describe.

• Understand that nourishment, which is the foundation of health, takes place on many levels, the most obvious of which is the physical. When we are well nourished by good-quality food, we will have good-quality health. But it doesn't end there. Nourishment is also to be found in the emotional, mental, and spiritual realms.

• Go back to nature. The principles of self-healing are revealed in nature, and they are fully accessible to us if we will only open our eyes to see them. Cycles of birth and death and re-birth, of balance and imbalance, of decline and self-repair, of seasonal changes, of light and darkness—all are apparent in nature, and all are part of the healing story. Getting in touch with nature is getting in touch with health.

> *It is important to* know *how to take care of ourselves so that we are free of the pains, aches, and acute ailments that may ulti-mately develop into chronic and degenerative diseases. . . . We cannot expect the tissues in our body to remain in a state of opti-mum health unless we have an evolved way of living, which springs from knowledge and wisdom.*
>
> Bernard Jensen, in Christopher Hobbs, *Foundations of Health,* 1992

> *I wish to present the truth in a practical manner, to help the*
> *human family, and to prevent others from becoming slaves to er-*
> *roneous ideas, so that mothers and fathers may better care for*
> *their families. . . .*
>
> *I wish to bring to the notice of the general public the*
> *untold blessings that our Heavenly Father has provided for*
> *all the world. It can be truly said, "My people are destroyed for*
> *lack of knowledge" (Hosea 4:6). A lack of knowledge based on*
> *truth is accountable for much of the untold sufferings and*
> *miseries of humanity.*
>
> Jethro Kloss, in *Back to Eden,* 1939

First Aid—with Nature

A few years ago in Albuquerque, Dr. Parcells was working late
in her office. Around midnight she heard someone stumbling up
her front steps. She went out on the porch to investigate and found
her neighbor trying to reach her door.

He was in terrible pain. "I dropped a battery and got the acid in
my eyes," he said. "I can't see, and I can't get help."

She led him to a sofa, where he could lie down, and remem-
bered that she had some heavy whipping cream in her refrigerator.
She poured some of the cream gently into his eyes and made a pack
with the rest of the cream and placed that over his eyes. He had been
in extreme agony, but within thirty minutes the pain was gone.

At that point Dr. Parcells sent her neighbor home with instructions to keep the cream pack on his eyes through the night, which
would lend relief until he could get to a doctor. The next morning
he went to see a doctor. By that time he had no pain at all and no

evidence of the dreadful accident. The doctor couldn't find any scarred tissue.

Within arm's reach, right in our own homes, we have many perfectly harmless materials to help us heal the body. These natural materials often do much more good than substances foreign to the body like pharmaceutical lotions and ointments.

Dr. Parcells knew that cream, which is fat, is part of the body's requirement. She also understood the simple chemistry of both sides of the problem—the biting, eating action of battery acid and the viscosity of the fat in cream, which would float any residue out. When applied to the eyes damaged by acid, cream healed the condition in nature's way.

She had similar success using cream to remove sand and other abrasive materials from eyes. Once, again with heavy cream, she saved the eye of a man who had gotten a sliver of dried paint stuck onto the inside of his eyelid; she performed that simple emergency remedy in the presence of a doctor, who was recommending an operation.

Another battery acid story. Many years ago, in Los Angeles, Dr. Parcells was driving along a highway and was passed by a speeding automobile. A few minutes later she came upon the same car, turned over in the middle of the road. A woman was pinned inside the car with battery acid leaking onto her legs. The woman was screaming for help.

Dr. Parcells rushed out of her car and joined two men who had been in the accident but were unhurt. Immediately she asked them to get her some motor oil. She poured the motor oil over the woman's legs to stop the pain. The oil was an unguent on the legs, blocking the wound from further damage and starting the process of healing. The woman's legs were saved that day, and her skin suffered no scars.

When Dr. Parcells herself took a fall a few years ago, she sustained a deep cut on the scalp. She instructed the naturopathic doctor who was visiting her at the time to pour cayenne pepper directly into the wound. He did, and the bleeding stopped immediately. She made a poultice with cayenne pepper also and applied that to her scalp. By the time she got to the local clinic, the gash was well on its way to complete healing. The wound was stitched and, two weeks later when the stitches were removed, there was no scar.

Dr. Parcells often recommended quite ordinary things found around the house to take care of ailments. For people with ulcers, she suggested a drink made from equal parts ginger ale and heavy cream. The cream soothes the ulcer, and the ginger stimulates healing. Even bleeding ulcers have been known to heal with this treatment.

Apple cider vinegar appears in many of her home remedies. She suggested it as a tonic for digestion: a tablespoon in a glass of warm water before a meal. For those who felt a cold coming on, she recommended the same drink; apple cider vinegar raises the acid level in the body—a cold comes in on an alkaline field.

Therapeutic bathing with two cups of apple cider vinegar detoxifies and softens the skin, raises the acid level in the body, and relaxes the muscles.

The acid/alkaline balance in the body was a main subject of Dr. Parcells's research and her remedies. People who are always tired and sleepy, she observed, are in an alkaline field and age more quickly. People whose systems are in a slightly acidic field age less quickly and have more pep and drive. The vast majority of illnesses exist and thrive in an alkaline medium. Keep the body slightly acidic, she advised.

Some of nature's remedies used by Dr. Parcells include:

Lemon juice: Fresh-squeezed in the morning with hot water as a way to flush the gall bladder and liver. An antiseptic and digestive. Gargle for sore throat. Lemon and water through the day cleanses and slims.

Garlic: A clove a day to counter high blood pressure. At the first onset of a cold, garlic soup made with several cloves of fresh garlic in chicken broth. A tonic for the lungs. A diuretic and antiseptic. In a poultice for symptoms of arthritis.

Cranberries: In a sauce with all meals as a digestive. Contains several powerful digestive enzymes. Reduces cholesterol buildup in the arteries. Juice (with water) as a flush and tonic for the kidneys.

Flax seeds: For ailments of the colon, especially colitis. Grind two tablespoons of fresh flax seed in a spice or coffee grinder and eat before retiring. Soothes and heals the end portion of the colon. Also a digestive and a laxative. (Must be ground fresh and taken within thirty minutes—being left standing longer renders the seed meal ineffective and slightly toxic.)

Parsley: Make into a tea to lower blood pressure and to use as a diuretic, a kidney and blood purifier. Has been known to flush out gallstones. Liver cleanser. Deodorant for the breath. (Use only fresh parsley.)

Ginger: Powdered ginger root or fresh ginger will address motion sickness. As a digestive and stimulant to assimilation. In a tea with honey and lemon for coughs and colds. Warms the stomach. Stops diarrhea. Good for bronchial problems.

Cornstarch: For diarrhea, ½ teaspoon in a glass of warm water; repeat if needed.

Salt: For hypoglycemia, ½ teaspoon in a glass of warm water. Also helpful for a "fading" feeling between meals: if blood sugar is too high, it will come down; if it is too low, it will come up. As an antidote for discomfort from sweet foods (salt counteracts the effects of sweetness; sweets, such as fresh fruits, counteract the effects of saltiness).

Baking soda: ½ teaspoon in a glass of warm water to neutralize stomach acid and bring the acid/alkaline level into balance. For nausea. Soaking foods in a solution of 1 tablespoon to 1 gallon of water will neutralize the effects of radiation and cobalt 60. For therapeutic bathing to release residues from X rays and other dangerous levels of radiation.

Apples: For constipation, one before retiring with a glass of water. A slice on a mosquito bite will stop the pain and itching and help heal the bite. As a cleanser for the internal organs. Boosts the immune system.

Olive oil (extra virgin, cold pressed): For dry skin, soak in hot tub with 2 tablespoons of olive oil. Moisturizes and lubricates skin, softening wrinkles. Good as natural nourishment for hair and nails. Full of potassium and phosphorus. Can dissolve gallstones. Lowers blood pressure, retards aging, reduces level of LDL ("bad") cholesterol and raises HDL ("good") cholesterol. Fights heart disease and cancer.

Water temperature: Cold-water soak of specific limbs for tendinitis. Take food supplements with warm or hot water for quickest assimilation.

THE MIRACLE OF THE PENDULUM

Of all the tools for self-help in health left to us by our ancestors, the pendulum may be the most important and the most valuable. It is probably also the simplest tool in the world. What could be less complicated than a string with a weight at the end of it?

Through the ages, people have used pendulums for all kinds of purposes, especially for divining and dousing. Dr. Parcells used pendulums to measure energy—mostly in matters related to health—but she was also able to assess the compatibility of persons, evaluate difficult situations, locate water, oil, and minerals, find missing items, detect earthquake activity, and engage them in many other applications.

One of her great legacies to us is her use of pendulum readings to determine the nutritional qualities of foods and their compatibility with each individual's chemical makeup. Another is her way of evaluating general health by using the pendulum to find places in the body where energy is needed to restore well-being.

> *The pendulum, properly used, is a scientific instrument. It is neither a toy nor a plaything. Those who know the laws of the pendulum hold the key to the universe in their hands.*
>
> Dr. Hazel Parcells

WHAT IS A PENDULUM?

The dictionary defines a pendulum as a body suspended from a fixed point that swings freely to and fro under the force of gravity. For our purposes, a pendulum is a weight suspended from a string held between the thumb and index finger; its movements indicate positive or negative energies.

In the 1950s, when she headed the school of nutrition at Sierra States University, Dr. Parcells worked with a European scientist to design a pendulum that would take the most accurate measurements of energy. The pendulum she developed was about four inches long and made of stainless steel, with a silver-coated chain suspended from a small loop. She used this pendulum in all her research, for forty years accurately measuring the energy in foods and in the human body.

The pendulum designed by Dr. Parcells is inexpensive and available from Parcells Center.

You can also make your own pendulum: a small crystal suspended from a thread, a cork into which you stick a needle and thread, a heavy button hung from a thin string—any of these crude versions of pendulums will give you positive/negative energy readings.

Proper Use of the Pendulum

To begin:

- Turn off the television, radio, or stereo; sounds carry energy— the pendulum will pick it up and measure it.

- Remove all jewelry from your hands and arms, especially rings and watches.

- Sit at a table or desk of comfortable height. Avoid working on metal surfaces, because metal will influence the energy readings.

- Place yourself in a listening attitude and disengage your mind. Don't think, just observe.

- Hold the pendulum in your right hand (in the left if you are left-handed) by placing your thumb and index finger together, loosely "pinching" the string or chain from which the weight hangs.

- Tuck your other three fingers into your palm so they won't act as antennas and attract unwanted energy that will alter your reading. (Notice if and how the pendulum's swing is affected when you increase or lessen the pressure of your thumb and index finger—just observe).

- Keep your legs uncrossed, feet on the floor, elbow in, out, or anchored on the table or the arm of a chair.

Now you're ready to get pendulum readings. The pendulum provides information in three ways:

1. Movement to the right, or clockwise motion, means positive, or "yes."

2. Movement to the left, or counterclockwise motion, means negative, or "no."

3. Movement back and forth means neutral, or "unknown at this time," or "no attraction."

With the pendulum in your right hand, hold your left hand out in front of you with the palm up (reverse hands if you are left-handed). Separate your fingers a bit. Hold the pendulum about an inch above the tip of the third finger on the outstretched hand. In a moment you should get a clockwise reading—the middle finger has a positive energy charge.

Now try the index finger. You should get a counterclockwise reading—the index finger has a negative energy charge.

Your thumb is neutral. You should get a back-and-forth swing of the pendulum.

The pendulum operates on the principle of opposites. "Yes" and "No" have their counterparts in nature, and form the basis of many systems of energetic healing, including Oriental medicine. These are the manifestations of opposites, used as part of Traditional Chinese Medicine.

Yang	Yin

In the natural world:

Day	Night
Clear day	Cloudy day
Spring/summer	Autumn/winter
East/south	West/north
Hot	Cold
Fire	Water
Light	Dark
Sun	Moon

In the body:

Surface of body	Interior of body
Spine/back	Chest/abdomen
Male	Female

Felix Mann, M.B., in *Acupuncture,* 1962

Using the Pendulum to Assess Compatibility with Foods

No two people are affected in the same way by the same food. Even in the same family, one person may be able to tolerate a diet that includes heavy proteins like red meat, while another may find the digestion of red meat next to impossible. Nutrition is a personal science, and each person's requirement is different. Using the pendulum is one way to obtain daily guidance in the selection of foods.

You can design your own special eating programs with the pendulum. Finding out which foods will enhance health *for you* and which foods will detract from *your* health will allow you always to select and eat the right foods for your body.

Give your pendulum an outing on this list. With the pendulum in one hand, use the other to point to each of these foods with a wooden chopstick. See what you come up with.

APPLES

RED MEAT

POPCORN

SPINACH

WHOLE WHEAT BREAD

BROWN RICE

PIZZA

PEANUTS

CARROTS

WHITE SUGAR

FISH

HONEY

Foods that gave you a positive reading are ones to include in your diet; foods that read negative should be avoided—you don't digest them properly, and they will cause health problems for you at some point. (By the way, very few people can digest and assimilate popcorn.)

Sometimes you'll notice that the pendulum swings stronger and faster or weaker and slower with certain measurements. These enthusiastic or lethargic movements indicate degrees of positive or negative energy. If you get a "weak" positive reading for whole-wheat bread, include it in your regular eating—but not much of it.

See Appendix II for a full food chart to use with the pendulum.

Shopping with a Pendulum

Many people believe that the day will come—and may not be too far off—when pendulums will be as common a sight in super-markets as shopping carts and checkout stands.

You don't have to be a specialist in the science of the pendulum to use it for one of our most important activities—shopping for food.

- Check the life-energy in foods: at the produce bin, for in-stance, hold the pendulum over fruits or vegetables one at a time to get the strongest possible readings.

- Check the freshness of foods: the pendulum will respond the most positively to foods that are the freshest.

- "Is this good for *me*?" Holding the food in one hand and the pendulum in the other over the food item, discover whether it will add to your body's energy and general health.

Note: Try to keep your mind clear of emotions while operating the pendulum. Avoid asking it questions, even for "yes" or "no" an-swers.

When pointing to a food or the name of a food, use a wooden chopstick. It will separate your body's energy from the energy being measured and give a truer reading.

The pendulum is a tool for communicating with the deeper, more hidden levels of our being, the part of us that is, unfortunately, clouded by fear, ignorance, and false-to-fact opinions about ourselves and the universe we live in, the part of us that knows the truth because it is the truth. These levels of being are not conditioned by space and time and have powers that we as humans have not even begun to understand.

Greg Nielsen and Joseph Polansky, in *Pendulum Power,* 1977

Recommended Reading on the Pendulum

Askew, Stella. *How to Use a Pendulum.* Mokelumne Hill, CA: Health Research, 1955.

Lethbridge, T. C. *The Power of the Pendulum.* London: Routledge and Kegan Paul; Boston: Henley, 1976.

MacDonald, Howard Breton. *The Pendulum Speaks.* Ontario: Provoker Press, 1969.

Nielsen, Greg, and Joseph Polansky. *Pendulum Power.* Rochester, VT: Destiny Books, 1977.

Strutt, Malcolm. *The Theory and Practice of Using the Pendulum.* London: Centre Community Publications, 1971.

This short list was chosen from a much longer list of seventy-four books and periodicals on the subject—with the use of a pendulum.

The Pendulum and Allergies

As you become more sophisticated in your use of the pendulum, you can begin to find out more about what's going on inside you. Take allergies, for instance. For twenty-five to thirty million people in the United States, allergies present a real health problem. An allergic reaction is a way our bodies reject something incompatible with its proper functioning. Almost any substance can become an *allergen*—something our immune system mistakes for a harmful invader.

Allergies fall into three different categories:

Contact allergies—caused by such things as perfumes, drugs, or clothing

Food allergies—reactions to specific foods (common ones are dairy products, shellfish, and corn)

Airborne and inhalant allergies—induced by substances such as pollen

Fully 15 percent of the American public suffers from allergies and treats them with common, over-the-counter drugs, whether prescribed or simply picked from the shelves of drugstores or supermarkets. These remedies treat symptoms temporarily but can often have unwanted and health-compromising side effects.

Antihistamines cause drowsiness and depress the immune system. Oral decongestants can cause insomnia and contribute to high blood pressure. Injections of drugs that control allergies are invasive and require adherence to a grueling regime: two shots a week for the first eight to sixteen weeks, then weekly shots after that for perhaps a year and more.

The answer to the problem of allergic reactions is the obvious one: avoid those things that bring on the reaction. The trouble is, we don't always know what is causing the problem.

Using the pendulum, you can discover the cause of an allergic reaction by going down a list of "suspects." It is easy to get "yes" and "no" responses to pendulum plumbing.

Pointing to items on a list with a wooden chopstick in one hand while holding a pendulum in the other and watching the pendulum's movement can pinpoint a potential troublesome substance.

Self-Appraisal: Food Supplements

If you want to know exactly which vitamins, minerals, or other supplements you should take to stay in good health, it's better not to guess—or worse, take the advice of advertisements in health magazines.

Try using the pendulum to ascertain what you truly need and the dosages appropriate for you. Readings may vary from day to day or from week to week, but that's normal, since our bodies change with the quality of food taken into it and the amount of energy expended.

If you are using a picture of a food supplement or the name of the supplement written in pencil on plain white paper, remember to use a wooden chopstick to point to the item when allowing the pendulum to make the determination.

A note about food supplements: Generally, Dr. Parcells believed that we should obtain full nourishment from the food we eat, but she did see the value in mineral supplements and antioxidants. Contact Parcells Center for recommendations on supplements.

Parcells Center
P.O. Box 2129
Santa Fe, NM 87504–2129
1–800–811–6784

ENERGY DISTORTION

Once you've gained experience with the pendulum, you can experiment with a healing technique to treat what

Dr. Parcells called "energy distortion." She used this as part of her regular method of helping others.

Every injury to the human body causes a release and loss of either positive or negative energy. In minor injuries, the loss is quickly healed. In severe injuries, the loss creates an imbalance in the cells, and so-called disease is the result. If we can stop the loss of "leaking" energy and return that energy back to the body, health is restored.

The greatest instrument in the world for healing is the human hand. The healer's body is a receptor of energy, and that energy is transmitted through the body and directed by and through the finger to the exact location of the energy distortion causing dis-ease or pain in another person's body. The pendulum locates the exact spot on the surface of the body where the energy distortion exists. The pendulum swings clockwise or counterclockwise according to the type of energy lost at that point. Directing the proper energy into the distortion will correct the energy loss.

- Locate the "energy distortion" by slowly moving your pendulum across the area of the body involved. The pendulum will swing back and forth (neutral) if normal energy is present. When an energy distortion is found, the pendulum will move in either a positive (clockwise) or negative (counterclockwise) direction.

- Once you have located the distortion, apply the appropriate energy emanating from your finger tips to the affected area: simply point about an inch away—the index finger (negative energy) if the escaping energy is negative, the middle finger (positive energy) if the escaping energy is positive.

- Continue working until you receive a neutral reading all over the affected area.

Think of energy in the body as blood. If someone punctures the skin, blood will flow out. Energy flows out of the body in the same way. We can stop bleeding with a bandage; we can stop an energy leak by applying our own energy to the place where there is an "energy distortion."

Say a child has fallen on the sidewalk and scraped his knee. The knee is the affected area. With your pendulum in your hand, get a neutral reading from the unaffected part of the leg. Then move the pendulum over the affected area until you begin to get a positive or negative reading. If the reading is positive, then positive energy is escaping from the wound. Point your own positive energy (from the middle finger of your other hand) above the affected area until your pendulum begins to register a neutral reading. If the reading is negative (meaning that negative energy is escaping from the child's body), apply energy from your index finger.

> *If you came to me with a gash in your arm, I would use an elementary method to heal the "energy distortion," as it is called. This natural technique makes healers of us all.*
>
> *When the skin of a worker's fingertips had been cut off in an accident, I put it back on using the natural energy from my own body; in an hour the man was back on the job. Out camping once, one of our party got his thumb caught in the door of the car. I cleaned away the blood, applied the same method to the energy distortion, and he was back to normal in a few minutes.*
>
> *A child of three and a half was riding her tricycle toward me. Her foot got caught in the pedals and twisted, and she fell flat onto the sidewalk. With the method of treating the energy distortion I had learned, I used the energy from*

> *my body to stop the flow of energy out of her scrapes and*
> *cuts; fifteen minutes later the child was up and playing*
> *again.*
>
> Dr. Hazel Parcells

THE HEALING CONSCIOUSNESS

The healing consciousness is aware of pulsating life all around and in every living being. It profoundly understands that health is our birthright as children of this planet. From that wellspring of knowing, animated by gratitude, radiates a healing energy that we can own and impart to other people.

WHAT YOU CAN DO TODAY
FOR BETTER HEALTH

· Increase your personal inventory of knowledge about the human body and how it works—read, study, and experiment with natural self-healing methods.

· Share health: resolve to extend your knowledge about health to others, knowing that the "circle of healing" will be most effective when healing is shared.

· Learn how to use simple foods and condiments for good health and especially how to treat emergency health situations.

· Master the use of the pendulum for assessment of your own and others' health problems.

Afterword

Beyond Nutrition

We work all our days building our life—and to what end? I believe it is, finally, to give it away to others. By this means, our life becomes a seed. Planted in the imagination of one who is ready to receive it, harbor it, and nourish it, the seed becomes the life of the future.

DR. HAZEL PARCELLS

A DEEPER LOOK AT NOURISHMENT

You know, I'm not a religious person," Dr. Parcells said one summer day while we were sitting out on the porch at Sapello, looking out at the mountains. "But I do believe I am a deeply spiritual person."

It was the first time since I had met her a year earlier that I'd heard her speak about such things. She went on to explain the difference between religion and spirituality. So many wars have been fought through the centuries in the name of religion, she said. So much killing, so many atrocities that are affronts to nature have been perpetrated to try to establish one belief system over another. These have been conducted by religious people. All of them believed they had God on their side. But spirituality had very little to do with any of it.

Dr. Parcells drew much of her sustenance from the spiritual side of life. It certainly was as important to her personally as any food regime or health-promoting habits she followed.

Many things nourish us; food is only one of those things.

This book focuses mainly on the physical body—how to clean it inside and out, how to nourish it, and how to keep it healthy all the days of our lives. However, total health goes far beyond merely the physical, into realms we can't see with the eye, hear with the ear, or feel with the fingertip.

EMOTIONAL "FOOD"

Emotional sustenance is an area of inquiry that is just now beginning for people who study nutrition. The simple premise is that there is an emotional counterpoint to food and it relates directly to physical well-being. To be truly fed and truly satisfied, more is necessary for us than food and drink; what is needed is "emotional food."

Imagine in the future a book about "emotional nutrition." It would warn you against all the toxic feelings that are out there in the world; advise you on how to purge and rejuvenate your emotional body; warn you against picking up other people's poisonous feelings; develop in you a sense of responsibility for your own emotions; and encourage you to help others heal themselves from emotional malfunctions.

When Dr. Parcells said, "we are overfed and undernourished," she meant it on many different levels. She meant it, in fact, to apply to the totality of what we are—physical, emotional, psychological, spiritual. In the emotional realm, we do seem to be bombarded with "stuff"—just take a look at the TV evening news or the programming that follows it. Whether any of it nourishes our emotional life is rather doubtful. Some popular entertainment has been called "junk food for the eyes," which is an apt description of so many elements in our culture that are designed as distractions.

Total nourishment includes emotional feeding. If that part of us is neglected, we're out of balance and therefore a sitting target for illness.

Some recommendations for emotional nutrition:

- Say "I love you" to a friend—and mean it, feel it. Expressing feelings of love brings about healing (there are statistics to prove it) in both the person receiving those expressions and the person articulating them. Men, particularly, can benefit from this form of emotional nutrition. Express love freely, lavishly, and unconditionally.

- Receive love. Feelings of unworthiness may have crept into your emotional life, but accepting love, embracing the feeling of being loved, is one of the ways to dispel those feelings. Accept away! It's nourishing.

- Hug. Physical touch connects us with others. It may be difficult for us in today's culture to touch and hug, but the therapeutic value of doing so has been proven clinically (children who are not hugged often are prone to illness). Hugging is good for health.

- Express your emotions—that's what they're there for. Unexpressed emotions are like undigested food: they build up in you like toxic wastes and create a health problem.

> *If scientists suddenly discovered a drug that was as powerful as love in creating health, it would be heralded as a medical breakthrough and marketed overnight—especially if it had as few side effects and was as inexpensive as love. Love is intimately related with health. This is not sentimental exaggeration. One survey of ten thousand men with heart disease found a 50 percent reduction in frequency of chest pain (angina) in men who perceived their wives as supportive and loving.*
>
> Larry Dossey, M.D., in *Healing Words*, 1993

OUR THOUGHTS CREATE OUR WORLD

If you are to be truly healthy, thought should be given to thought; that is, what you think is as important as what you do. An attitude that regards plants and animals and the rest of nature as inferior to human beings is arrogant, and such thoughts will boomerang back upon us with tenfold force.

"Species arrogance," or speciesism, is what has gotten us into so much trouble in the past century. We killed off vast stretches of nature to increase our human food supply—and we ended up killing each other. And, if all the doomsday environmental warnings are correct, we're in the process of killing ourselves also.

Psychological health relates to thinking thoughts that bring about oneness over separation, serenity and assurance over fear, perception over confusion, and healing over disease. We are what we think as surely as we are what we eat. If our thinking is out of balance with what is patently obvious from nature as the principles of life, we'll suffer the consequences in our bodies.

For nourishment on the psychological level:

- Regard all life as precious, important, and worthy of continuing in existence. All life includes you as a living being, of course, so taking an embracing attitude toward life brings you back, full circle, to self-acceptance.

> *Chronic stomach trouble is most frequently found among the worriers and those whose delicate egos are easily bruised. Nervous stomach trouble is a difficult ailment to bear gracefully, but if the mind can be directed to become less critical of others, more tolerant in its viewpoints, the digestion will immediately show a marked improvement.*
>
> *While all sickness cannot be traced to disposition, it can be said with accuracy that all persons with bad dispositions are sick. A bad disposition is one of the heaviest burdens that the flesh can bear.*
>
> Manly P. Hall, in *Healing, the Divine Art*, 1972

- "Think no evil." Understand that directing venomous thoughts at someone or something can make you ill. It works on the principle of oneness, or karma: what you will for another is done to you, since we all share life and therefore are one. To be healthy, think good thoughts.

- Don't judge. Judgment is a prison you make for everyone and everything that receives it. When you judge people, you imprison them in a small box of thought; they react according to your determination of them. The same is true of situations. Avoiding judgment is the foundation of healing others and the assurance of good health for yourself.

SPIRITUAL HEALTH

Our relationship to something greater than ourselves—a Supreme Being, a Great Spirit, God, the Higher Self—is the end, and the beginning, of health. There simply can be no true and lasting health on the physical, emotional, and psychological planes if no attention is given to a sense of the Divine.

The reason the spiritual dimension needs to be included in matters of health should be obvious: all of nature, all of life, is evidence of the workings of a Higher Power (since we ourselves didn't bring life into being); not to acknowledge that Power in some way points to an imbalance—and, as we've seen, being out of balance is one definition of illness.

In some cultures in ages past, sickness was equated with having a spiritual problem. From witch doctors to medicine men to the cult of Asclepius in ancient Greece, out of which tradition came Hippocrates, the father of medicine, healers have looked to spiritual causes for physical maladies.

They did so not from ignorance, but from a profound understanding of the spiritual nature of all life. Only recently, as human history goes, have we divorced spirit from the material world, trying to make sense of the parts of the cosmic drama without taking into account the whole of it.

"God tolerates atheists," Dr. Parcells used to say. However, nature has a harder time with them. If you will be healthy all the time, which is to say, if you will be whole, seek out and cultivate the spiritual foundation of life.

Some suggestions:

• Be still. It's also called meditation. This is not a religious activity, but a spiritual one. In the words of an old sage, "Prayer is us talking to God—meditation is God talking to us." Meditation is the state of receptivity. The wonderful thing about meditation is that you don't have to *do* anything. You just sit quietly, letting go of your thoughts and letting the power of the Universe in.

• Forgive. The spiritual book *A Course in Miracles*, which Marianne Williamson wrote about, says, "All disease comes from a state of unforgiveness; whenever we are ill, we need to look around to see who it is that we need to forgive." Forgiving is releasing another (or yourself) from anything you believe is owing to you. Releasing freely will result in good and lasting health.

• Appreciate, and be grateful. Sincere gratitude unlocks every other door to healing that may have been closed to you. It is an acknowledgment of the generosity, beauty, joy, and abundance of life.

• Surrender and trust. Imagine yourself as a sleeping child in the arms of a loving parent. You were given life; it is a gift. Trusting in the Giver of Life to move nature to its perfect unfoldment— and you to yours—invites into your experience the miracle of health.

Appendix I

The Parcells Detoxification and Rejuvenation Program

The Parcells Detoxification and Rejuvenation Program is a carefully structured eight-day plan designed to cleanse the body *at the cell level* of stored toxins. It was developed by Dr. Parcells over a decade of scientific research on body chemistry.

- Read all instructions carefully before beginning the program.

- The Cell Cleanse powder should be used *only* while on the program.

- All juices should be fresh, not frozen, if possible, and unsweetened.

- Avoid using canned juices—fresh-squeezed juices in glass or plastic containers will give best results.

- Drink as much water as you desire—at least six 8-ounce glasses of water per day.

Used in the program are the Parcells Cell Cleanse and the Parcells Natural Regulator. The Cell Cleanse powder contains dandelion root, parsley root, yellowdock root, thyme, celery seed, horseradish, cayenne pepper, slippery elm, and cranberry powder in a compound created by Dr. Parcells to exact specifications for the most effective cleansing at the cell level.

The ingredients in the Natural Regulator powder include kelp, rhubarb root, slippery elm, sena leaf, cascara sagrada, cranberry powder, dulce powder, and ground flax seed in proportions developed by Dr. Parcells as an eliminator and colon conditioner over many years of research.

Both the Cell Cleanse and the Natural Regulator needed to do this program are available at the present time only through:

Parcells Center
P.O. Box 2129
Santa Fe, NM 87504–2129

INSTRUCTIONS FOR PREPARING THE CELL CLEANSE

Prepare enough Cell Cleanse for an entire day. Allow 1 rounded teaspoon of the Cell Cleanse powder for each 8 ounces of liquid. When the Cell Cleanse is to be taken 6 times daily, use 6 rounded teaspoons of the Cell Cleanse powder, add 3 cups of boiling water, stir thoroughly, and add 3 cups tomato juice. Mix well. This may be taken hot or cold, as desired. *Do not use aluminum containers.*

DAILY SCHEDULE

N*ote:* the starting time given is meant as a guide; if you begin later than 7:00 A.M. each day, simply calculate everything from your starting hour.

Copy out the following pages and use them as a checklist as you go through the program.

Days One, Two, and Three

_____7 A.M.	*Morning tonic: 4 oz. sauerkraut and 4 oz. tomato juice pureed together in a blender*
_____8 A.M.	*8 oz. Cell Cleanse, with 1 tsp. Natural Regulator added*
_____9 A.M.	*8 oz. grapefruit juice*
_____10 A.M.	*8 oz. Cell Cleanse*
_____11 A.M.	*8 oz. grapefruit juice*
_____12 noon	*8 oz. Cell Cleanse*
_____1 P.M.	*8 oz. grapefruit juice*
_____2 P.M.	*8 oz. Cell Cleanse*
_____3 P.M.	*8 oz. grapefruit juice*
_____4 P.M.	*8 oz. Cell Cleanse*
_____5 P.M.	*8 oz. grapefruit juice*
_____6 P.M.	*8 oz. Cell Cleanse with 1 tsp. Natural Regulator added*
_____7 P.M.	*8 oz. grapefruit juice*

Before retiring on the third day, the Liver Cleanse (see below).

Days Four and Five

_____	7 A.M.	*Morning tonic: 4 oz. sauerkraut and 4 oz. tomato juice pureed together in a blender*
_____	8 A.M.	*8 oz. Cell Cleanse with 1 tsp. Natural Regulator added*
_____	9 A.M.	*8 oz. grapefruit juice*
_____	10 A.M.	*8 oz. Cell Cleanse*
_____	11 A.M.	*8 oz. apple juice*
_____	12 noon	*8 oz. Cell Cleanse*
_____	1 P.M.	*8 oz. grapefruit juice*
_____	2 P.M.	*8 oz. Cell Cleanse*
_____	3 P.M.	*8 oz. apple juice*
_____	4 P.M.	*8 oz. Cell Cleanse*
_____	5 P.M.	*8 oz. grapefruit juice*
_____	6 P.M.	*8 oz. apple juice*
_____	7 P.M.	*8 oz. Cell Cleanse with 1 tsp. Natural Regulator added*

Before retiring on the fifth day, the Liver Cleanse (see below).

Days Six and Seven

_____	7 A.M.	*Morning tonic: 4 oz. sauerkraut and 4 oz. tomato juice pureed together in a blender*
_____	8 A.M.	*8 oz. Cell Cleanse with 1 tsp. Natural Regulator added*
_____	9 A.M.	*8 oz. apple juice*
_____	10 A.M.	*8 oz. fresh fruit, in season if possible (one kind)*

_____11 A.M.	8 oz. Cell Cleanse	
_____12 noon	8 oz. fresh fruit (one kind)	
_____1 P.M.	8 oz. Cell Cleanse	
_____2 P.M.	8 oz. apple juice	
_____3 P.M.	fresh fruit (one kind, any quantity)	
_____4 P.M.	8 oz. Cell Cleanse	
_____5 P.M.	8 oz. apple juice	
_____6 P.M.	fresh fruit (one kind, any quantity)	
_____7 P.M.	8 oz. Cell Cleanse with 1 tsp. Natural Regulator added	

Note: Use any fresh fruit except bananas and citrus fruits.

Day Eight

_____7 A.M.	Morning tonic: 4 oz. sauerkraut and 4 oz. tomato juice pureed together in a blender
_____8 A.M.	8 oz. Cell Cleanse with 1 tsp. Natural Regulator added
_____9 A.M.	8 oz. apple juice
_____10 A.M.	fresh fruit (one kind, any quantity)
_____11 A.M.	8 oz. Cell Cleanse
_____12 noon	LUNCH: One bunch of parsley (fresh or steamed) or ½ lb. asparagus or 1 bunch of spinach steamed (use only fresh vegetables). If desired, add a sprinkle of salt and a small amount of butter or olive oil.

Repeat the lunch meal for dinner, with the addition of a cooked or raw fruit in season.

Upon retiring take 1 tsp. Natural Regulator in 8 oz. apple juice. Repeat for several days after completing the program upon retiring.

THE LIVER CLEANSE

Mix together 4 oz. grapefruit juice and 4 oz. extra virgin olive oil to form an emulsion, and drink it.

Lie quietly on the *right* side for 15 or 20 minutes to avoid nausea.

Drink 8 oz. grapefruit juice.

Retire, lying on the *right* side.

The next morning, watch the stool for small, green pellets sometimes as large as birds' eggs. This is waste material from the gall bladder, a sign that you are freeing yourself of deeply stored toxins.

THE INTERNAL BATH

Many people who have gone through the program have benefited by including the internal bath or a colonic once or twice daily, morning and evening. It is recommended that you do the internal bath at least three times during the program.

For the internal bath, mix 1 tablespoon blackstrap molasses in 1 quart warm water and use an enema.

A colonic, or deep cleaning of the colon, is an excellent way to assist the internal cleansing process. Ask your health care professional to recommend someone in your area who is trained to perform colonics.

THERAPEUTIC BATHING

Therapeutic baths can be used to release accumulated toxins through the skin, the largest eliminative organ of your body, enhancing the cleansing process.

Any one or more of the four Parcells therapeutic baths listed in Step Two may be included in the program. Therapeutic bathing should be done in the evening, before retiring. Use only one bath per evening and follow the directions to the letter.

FOOD DURING AND FOLLOWING
THE PROGRAM

Use only foods listed above during the eight days of the cleansing program. Any fresh fruit in season may be used *except bananas and citrus fruits*. Only one kind of fruit should be eaten at one time, but in any quantity desired.

For the first two days after the cleansing program has been completed, it's best to refrain from eating grain starches, such as bread, cereals, rice, and pasta. Also, avoid all sugar and pastries. Eat light meals. To satisfy hunger between meals, eat fresh green vegetables and fresh fruits in any quantity.

For optimum assimilation of quality, high-energy food at this time, refer to the recommendations on food cleaning and food combining in Step Three and Step Four.

PROGRAM SHOPPING LIST

Note: All juices should be in *plastic* or *glass containers,* not cans.

Tomato juice	*6¼ quarts*
Grapefruit juice	*7⅛ quarts (includes juice for the Liver Cleanse)*
Apple juice	*5 quarts (will provide for 6 evening laxatives following the cleanse)*

Sauerkraut	*1 quart*
Fruit	*4½ pounds (more if desired), fresh, in season*
Cell Cleanse	*from Parcells Center*
Natural Regulator	*from Parcells Center*

A timer, if you think you might have trouble remembering your hourly juice or broth.

TWENTY QUESTIONS

1. Will I be hungry on this program?

Most people never feel a bit of hunger. Some people feel some hunger on the first day. On the program, your body goes into an entirely different mode of intake and expenditure. Don't be alarmed if you feel a slight discomfort during the first day or two of the program. Remember, you are in the process of a major detoxification, and all those poisons are bound to make a little curtain call as they leave the stage forever.

2. Will I feel weak?

Not really. But you should give yourself ample rest during the program. If you feel like lying down a lot, do so. But take only catnaps to avoid missing your hourly juice or broth.

3. Should I exercise on the program?

It's better to exercise only lightly. A walk in the woods—or, if a woods is not nearby, a walk around the block—is probably enough to continue the detoxification process by gently stimulating the internal organs.

4. Can I drink coffee, tea, sodas, or any other liquid besides the water, juice, and broth specified in the program?

No. Caffeine drinks, especially, will throw off the chemistry of the program. Don't worry—your craving for caffeine will disappear in a short time.

5. How important is it to be on time with the hourly juice and broth?

It's vitally important to take the appropriate liquid at the appointed hour to avoid hunger and to assure the effectiveness of the cleansing. But you can adjust the *starting* hour according to your schedule. If you don't rise in the morning until 9:45, take the first (7:00) program feeding at 10:00—and then stay on an hourly schedule until 10:00 in the evening.

6. If I *don't* do the liver cleanses or internal baths, will I still get the full benefits of the program?

No, you won't. Do everything recommended here, including the liver cleanses and the internal baths. The therapeutic baths are highly recommended, but if you can only do one or two during the program, you will still be within the general recommendations.

7. Can I use canned fruit and vegetable juices?

No. Almost all canned juices come in aluminum cans—and aluminum is a strict no-no, because it is a health hazard.

8. Can I substitute vegetable juices like V-8 for the tomato juice?

No. The chemical constitutions are different.

9. How do I know if this program is for me?

Check with your health care professional before embarking on this program. It is a major detoxification program and should be taken seriously.

10. Can children go on this program?

Probably not. Again, check with your health care professional if there is any question.

11. Can elderly people go on this program?

Any adult in reasonably good health can do the program at any age. Dr. Parcells undertook the program every year or two well into her nineties.

12. Should I go on the program if I'm pregnant?

No. During pregnancy is not the best time to engage in detoxification. Some months before or some months after are better times.

13. I'm on prescription drugs for a number of health problems. Can I do this program and still take the drugs?

No. Drugs, including contraceptive pills, will compromise the chemical work of the program. Consult your health care professional to see whether you can stop taking the drugs during this wonderful cleansing adventure. If you can, chances are you will never need to go back on the drugs.

14. Can I just jump back into my old eating habits once I've completed the program?

No. But rest assured, you won't want to. You'll be so conscious of what you are putting into your body that you'll eat only what your body can use to build health. One thing this program brings about is a new awareness of food and its role in nutrition. Old cravings gradually will diminish.

15. Can I drink water on this program? If so, how much?

Water is highly recommended—at least six full 8-ounce glasses a day. Drink more if you feel hungry or thirsty. Water is the best flushing agent for toxins. Try to drink only clean, high-energy water while on the program; water cleaned and energized with full-spectrum lighting (see Step Three) will increase your body energy and promote faster detoxification and rejuvenation.

16. Will I be bored on this program?

That depends on you. If you feel yourself getting bored, read a good book—in fact, read this one again!

17. Can I eat anything I want once the program is over?

No. For the first two days after the program is complete, refrain from starchy foods, especially breads, pastas, and other grain products.

18. Will this program sap my energy?

On the contrary—it will enhance and increase your energy, as your body flushes out toxins and becomes more efficient at turning nourishment into energy. Most people report that by the fourth or fifth day they have so much energy that they have to moderate their activities so they won't overdo it.

19. How many times should I do this program?

Do it once. Then, a year later if you feel you would like to do it again, do so after consulting your health care professional. Subsequent repetitions of the program will be less dramatic—because your body has much less poison stored away in it.

20. How important are the emotional and psychological aspects of the cleansing program?

Extremely important! Monitor yourself for signs of old, toxic emotions or thought patterns emerging during the program. You'll see them, feel them, and find yourself letting them go—along with the physical toxins that are leaving your body.

Note: You may want to keep a journal while you are on the program. It helps to externalize your emotional and psychological states. Afterward, you'll be able to see real progress in this area.

If you have done the Parcells Detoxification and Rejuvenation Program once, you can do an abbreviated version of it at a later time. It's best to wait at least a few months before embarking on the shorter version. The general recommendation is to do this short version of the program every three months or so if you feel you need to clean house.

The shorter version: Days One, Two, and Three, as listed above. Follow the directions to the letter for those three days. Remember to include at least one liver cleanse, one internal bath, and one therapeutic bath; a colonic during this time is also a good idea.

This shorter version of the program is only for those who have done the full eight-day program at least once.

Appendix II

Food Chart for Use with the Pendulum

To help you determine which foods are likely to enhance health *for you*, here is a chart to use with your pendulum. Consult Step Six for particulars.

Hold your pendulum in your right hand (in the left if you are left-handed) and with the other point to each food listed here with a wooden chopstick. If you get a clockwise swing of the pendulum, the food should become part of your regular eating regime; if you get a counterclockwise swing, you should think about avoiding that particular food.

Beans and Legumes

black beans

black-eyed peas

garbanzos

kidney beans

lentils

lima beans

mung beans

navy beans

pinto beans

soybeans

split peas

Beverages

beer

coffee, decaf

coffee, regular

fruit juice

grain drink

liquor

milk, nut

milk, rice

milk, soy

mineral water

soda

soda, diet

tea, black

tea, green

tea, herbal

tea, yogi

vegetable juice

wine

Condiments

carob

catsup

cayenne

chilis, green

chilis, red

chocolate

cinnamon

cloves

curry

dill

dulse

garlic

gelatin

ginger

honey

horseradish

jello

jelly/jam

lard

margarine

mint

miso, barley

miso, soy

molasses

MSG

mustard

oil, canola

oil, corn

oil, olive

oil, peanut

oil, safflower

paprika

pepper, black

pepper, red

salsa

salt, iodized

salt, sea

salt, vegetable

seaweed

shortening

soy sauce

sugar, brown

sugar, white

syrup

vinegar

yeast

Dairy Products

butter

buttermilk

cheese, cheddar

cheese, cottage

cheese, cream

cheese, feta

cheese, Monterey jack

cheese, mozzarella

cheese, processed

cheese, Swiss

cream

ghee

ice cream

milk, goat

milk, skim

milk, whole

sherbet

sour cream

yogurt

yogurt, frozen

Fruits

apple

apricot

banana

black mulberry

blackberry

cantaloupe

cherry

cranberry

currant

date

fig

gooseberry

grape

grapefruit

honeydew

lemon

lime

nectarine

orange

papaya

peach

pear

persimmon

pineapple

plum

prune

raisin

raspberry, red

strawberry

tangerine

watermelon

Grains and Cereals

amaranth

barley

buckwheat

corn

crackers

millet

oats

pasta

quinoa

rice, basmati

rice, brown

rice, white

rice, wild

rye

spelt

wheat

wheat germ

Nuts and Seeds

almonds

Brazil nuts

cashews

coconut

flax seeds

hazelnuts

peanuts

pecans

pine nuts

pistachios

pumpkin seeds

sesame seeds

sunflower seeds

walnuts

Proteins

beef

chicken

clams

codfish

crab

duck

eggs

halibut

herring

lamb

lobster

mackerel

oysters

pork

rabbit

salmon

sardines

scallops

shrimp

tofu

trout

tuna

turkey

veal

whitefish

Vegetables

artichoke

asparagus

avocado	mushrooms
beet	okra
bell pepper	olives
broccoli	onion
Brussels sprouts	parsley
cabbage	parsnip
carrot	peas
cauliflower	popcorn
celery	potato
chips, corn	pumpkin
chips, potato	radish
chives	rhubarb
corn	spinach
cucumber	sprouts, bean
eggplant	squash
endive	string beans
escarole	sweet potato
garlic	Swiss chard
greens	tomato
kale	turnip
leeks	watercress
lettuce	yam

Index

About Parcells Center

Dr. Parcells founded Parcells Center to help others improve the quality of their lives by using her pioneering methods of natural self-healing. The center operates through a membership of people like you, who are taking responsibility for their health and looking for sound, reliable advice to help them.

A staff of dedicated professionals leads the center, networking with a large number of doctors and other experienced health specialists who are students and followers of Dr. Parcells, to service an ever-growing family of members.

The center is organized around four divisions: Education, Publications, Research, and Products. Education encompasses several programs, including classes in the Parcells Method at the center's headquarters in Santa Fe, New Mexico, and weekend workshops around the country. It conducts advanced courses in natural self-healing for health professionals and others seeking certification in the Parcells Method. It also directs a two-week rejuvenation retreat, where participants learn the principles of natural self-healing while engaging in a full detoxification and health-building regime.

The publications division produces the monthly *Parcells Letter*, which updates members on new discoveries from the Parcells Lab and from the Parcells Center Network. *The Parcells Letter* inspires and motivates members to improve the quality of their lives with practical applications of natural self-healing for today's health concerns. Publications also issues timely reports on a wide range of important health issues.

The research arm of Parcells Center extends the groundbreaking work of Dr. Parcells in developing hard data about dangers to health—and what can be done to restore well-being through drugless, noninvasive practices. The lab is constantly seeking new ways to understand the causes of physical disorders, and recommending natural remedies for them.

The Parcells products are vital tools for natural self-healing developed by Dr. Parcells herself, from food supplements to bath aids, from homeopathic remedies to home appliances. New products to meet new challenges to health are in continual development by the lab, networking with Parcells practitioners in the field.

MEMBERSHIP IN PARCELLS CENTER

To become a member of Parcells Center, and be part of a family that is deeply committed to your health, write or phone us:

Parcells Center
P.O. Box 2129
Santa Fe, NM 87504-2129
1-800-811-6784
e-mail: parcellscn@aol.com
Web site: www.parcellscenter.com